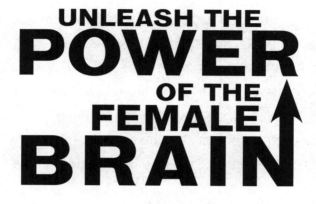

UNLEASH THE
POWER
OF THE
FEMALE
BRAIN

BOOKS BY DR. AMEN

USE YOUR BRAIN TO CHANGE YOUR AGE (Crown Archetype, 2012)

THE AMEN SOLUTION (Crown Archetype, 2011)

END OF EMOTIONAL OVEREATING (written with Larry Momaya, M.D., MindWorks, 2011)

UNCHAIN YOUR BRAIN (MindWorks, 2010)

WIRED FOR SUCCESS (MindWorks, 2010)

CHANGE YOUR BRAIN, CHANGE YOUR BODY (Harmony Books, 2010)

MAGNIFICENT MIND AT ANY AGE (Harmony Books, 2009)

THE BRAIN IN LOVE (Three Rivers Press, 2007)

MAKING A GOOD BRAIN GREAT (Harmony Books, 2005)

PREVENTING ALZHEIMER'S (written with neurologist William R. Shankle, Putnam, 2004)

HEALING ANXIETY AND DEPRESSION (written with Lisa Routh, M.D., Putnam, 2003)

NEW SKILLS FOR FRAZZLED PARENTS (MindWorks, 2003)

HEALING THE HARDWARE OF THE SOUL (Free Press, 2002)

IMAGES OF HUMAN BEHAVIOR: A BRAIN SPECT ATLAS (MindWorks, 2003)

HEALING ADD (Putnam, 2001)

HOW TO GET OUT OF YOUR OWN WAY (MindWorks, 2000)

CHANGE YOUR BRAIN, CHANGE YOUR LIFE (Three Rivers Press, 1999)

ADD IN INTIMATE RELATIONSHIPS (MindWorks, 1997)

WOULD YOU GIVE 2 MINUTES A DAY FOR A LIFETIME OF LOVE? (St. Martin's Press, 1996)

A CHILD'S GUIDE TO ADD (MindWorks, 1996)

A TEENAGER'S GUIDE TO ADD (written with Antony Amen and Sharon Johnson, MindWorks, 1995)

MINDCOACH: TEACHING KIDS TO THINK POSITIVE AND FEEL GOOD (MindWorks, 1994)

THE MOST IMPORTANT THING I LEARNED IN LIFE I LEARNED FROM A PENGUIN (MindWorks, 1994)

TEN STEPS TO BUILDING VALUES WITHIN CHILDREN (MindWorks, 1994)

THE SECRETS OF SUCCESSFUL STUDENTS (MindWorks, 1994)

HEALING THE CHAOS WITHIN (MindWorks, 1993)

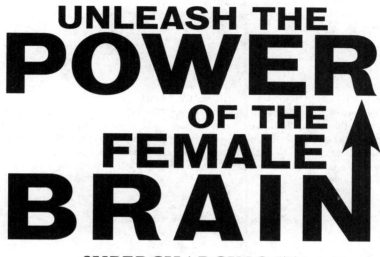

UNLEASH THE POWER OF THE FEMALE BRAIN

SUPERCHARGING IT FOR BETTER HEALTH, ENERGY, MOOD, FOCUS, AND SEX

Daniel G. Amen, M.D.

Uncorrected Proof

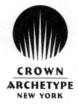

CROWN
ARCHETYPE
NEW YORK

MEDICAL DISCLAIMER

The information presented in this book is the result of years of practical experience and clinical research by the author. The information in this book, by necessity, is of a general nature and not a substitute for an evaluation or treatment by a competent medical specialist. If you believe you are in need of medical interventions please see a medical practitioner as soon as possible. The stories in this book are true. The names and circumstances of the stories have been changed to protect the anonymity of patients.

Published in the United States by Harmony Books, an imprint of the
Crown Publishing Group, a division of Random House, Inc., New York.
www.crownpublishing.com

Harmony Books and colophon are registered trademarks of Random House, Inc.

Library of Congress Cataloging-in-Publication Data

[CIP data]

ISBN 978–0-307–88894–5
eISBN 978–0-307–88896–9

Printed in the United States of America

Book design by
Illustrations by
Jacket design by
Jacket photography

10   9   8   7   6   5   4   3   2   1

First Edition

To the powerful women in my life!

My wife, Tana

My daughters, Breanne, Kaitlyn, and Chloe

My granddaughters, Angelina and Emmy

My mother, Dorie

My sisters, Chris, Jeanne, Mary, Renee, and Joanne

And my many aunts, nieces, grandnieces, and female cousins

CONTENTS

INTRODUCTION: THE FEMALE BRAIN UNLEASHED   000

1. FALL IN LOVE WITH YOUR FEMALE BRAIN: 000
   Care About Your Brain More Than Any Other Body Part

Hour 1 Exercise—Boost Brain Envy

**2. HARNESS THE UNIQUE STRENGTHS OF
THE FEMALE BRAIN:**   000
   *Use Your Intuition, Collaboration, Empathy, Self-Control,
   and a Little Worry to Give Yourself a Great Advantage*

Hour 2 Exercise—Recruit Your Team and Make Your
Worries Work for You

**3. ADOPT THE AMEN CLINICS' METHOD FOR OPTIMIZING
THE FEMALE BRAIN:**   000
   *Know Your Brain, Important Numbers, and
   the Four Circles for Ultimate Success*

Hour 3 Exercise—Get Assessed

**4. BALANCE YOUR HORMONES TO BOOST
THE FEMALE BRAIN**   000
   *Part One: Balance Estrogen, Progesterone, and
   Testosterone*
   Part Two: Balance Thyroid, Cortisol, DHEA, and Insulin

Hour 4 Exercise—Take the Hormone Questionnaires
and Inventory Your Healthy and Unhealthy Hormone
Habits

5. **FEED THE FEMALE BRAIN:** 000
*Flatten Your Tummy and Boost Brain Reserves by
Healing Your Gut and Eating Brain-Healthy Superfoods*

Hour 5 Exercise—Provide Therapy for Your Kitchen

6. **SOOTHE THE FEMALE BRAIN:** 000
*Put an End to Anxiety, Worry, Depression, and
Perfectionism*

Hour 6 Exercise—Get ANT Therapy and Answer the
Work's Four Questions

7. GET CONTROL OF THE FEMALE BRAIN:
Conquer Cravings, Weight Issues, and Addictions

Hour 7 Exercise—Embrace Your Failures

8. **UNDERSTAND ADD AND THE FEMALE BRAIN:** 000
*Learn to Treat the Hyperactive "Boys'" Condition That
Ruins Female Lives*

Hour 8 Exercise—Know Your Focus and Energy
Robbers and Boosters

9. **BE BEAUTIFUL ON THE INSIDE AND OUT:** 000
*Learn Strategies to Help Your Brain and Body Look
Amazing*

Hour 9 Exercise—Get a Massage and Enjoy a Sauna

10. **UNDERSTAND SEX AND THE FEMALE BRAIN:** 000
*Optimize Your Brain for Greater Pleasure, Deeper
Relationships, and Lasting Love*

Hour 10 Exercise—Be the Director of Your Pleasure

**11. GET YOUR BRAIN READY FOR BABIES AND
CARING FOR THEIR BRAINS ONCE THEY'RE HERE:** 000
*Prepare for Pregnancy—and Unleash the Power of
Your Daughters' Brains*

Hour 11 Exercise—Indulge in Special Time

12. CHANGE YOUR FEMALE BRAIN, CHANGE THE WORLD: 000
*Realize That It's Not AboutYou—It's About Generations
of You*

Hour 12 Exercise—Create Your Own Genius Network

**APPENDIX A: NATURAL SUPPLEMENTS TO HELP YOU UNLEASH
THE POWER OF YOUR FEMALE BRAIN** 000

NOTE ON REFERENCES 000

ACKNOWLEDGMENTS 000

INDEX 000

INTRODUCTION

THE FEMALE BRAIN UNLEASHED

I have an idea that the phrase "the weaker sex" was coined by some woman to disarm the man she was preparing to overwhelm.

—OGDEN NASH

My thought exactly. I have been surrounded by powerful women my whole life.

Growing up, there were so many women in my life that when my mother brought my fifth sister, Joanne, home from the hospital in December 1962, my older brother, Jimmy, and I ran away. Jimmy was nine and I was eight, and even though we were only gone for forty-five minutes, as the only boys, we had had enough! The girls had taken over and they were everywhere. I often joke that I never saw a bathroom until I was fourteen years old and that once I actually got in, there was unusual and frightening stuff scattered everywhere.

Not only was I was raised by a very powerful mother, who at eighty-one years old and five feet tall is still in charge everywhere she goes, but I have five strong-willed sisters, three incredible daughters, two granddaughters, and fourteen nieces and grandnieces. My wife says I came housebroken when it came to dealing with women, but it was not an easy process. As we will see, the female brain is very different from the male brain.

As I came to understand the complexity and power of the female brain, I marveled at what a difference this information could make to the experience of millions of women and to the men and children in their lives.

When a woman understands the uniqueness of the female brain—how to care for it, how to make the most of its strengths, how to overcome its challenges, how to fall in love with it, and ultimately, how to unleash its full power—there is no stopping her. In her personal development, at work, and in her relationships, she can bring the best of herself to her family, her community, and her planet.

By contrast, a woman who is not caring optimally for her brain, who is not giving it the full range of nutrients, exercise, sleep, and emotional support that it needs, is squandering her most valuable resource. If you are not taking good care of your brain, you are at a significantly higher risk of brain fog, memory problems, low energy, distractibility, poor decisions, obesity, heart disease, cancer, and diabetes. You can't have the vitality you need to get through the day with all the calm, focus, energy, and joy of which you are capable. You are most certainly going to age faster and become ill both more often and more seriously.

Those are the risks that both men and women share—but as a woman, you face some unique additional challenges. You are far more likely than a man to suffer from anxiety and depression and, in some studies, Alzheimer's disease. You are far more susceptible to recurring negative thoughts you just can't dismiss, to body image struggles that all too frequently morph into eating disorders, and to excessive self-criticism for not being perfect. You are also more prone to pouring yourself into the care of your loved ones and the demands of your job, your family, and your community, finding it ever more difficult to take the time you need to care for yourself.

These are the risks you face, but you don't have to fall prey to them. Caring for your female brain and learning how to unleash its power can free you to reach your full potential to be healthy, loving, successful, and strong. It can allow you to have more satisfying intimate relationships and make you a better partner. And it can make you a more effective person at your chosen work. For women who choose to have children, it also prepares you for a successful pregnancy and equips you to help your children fully unleash the power of *their* brains.

Unleashing the power of your female brain is your key to finally having the life you've dreamed of and deserve.

THE FEMALE BRAIN CAN CHANGE THE WORLD

With the epidemic escalation of obesity, diabetes, depression, and dementia, the health of Western society is going the wrong way at an ever increasingly rapid pace. Now more than ever, we need thoughtful, intelligent, powerful, "brain smart" women, to guide and redirect our families, communities, churches, workplaces, nation, and world. And women are in a unique position to make a dramatic difference.

One of the reasons I decided to write this book now is that I know what an enormous difference women can make. Growing up, my mother was the health leader in our home, and today my wife, Tana, plays the same role. I have seen this pattern repeat over and over in the families I treat as a physician. As the adult females take better care of themselves, it tends to positively affect those around them.

As a neuroscientist, psychiatrist, and brain imaging specialist, I have known for decades that women typically take their physical and mental health more seriously than men do. That is one of the reasons, I'm convinced, that they also live longer on average than men. In 2010, U.S. women lived an average of eighty years, as opposed to only seventy-three years for U.S. men. In Russia, women live twelve years longer than men—so, men, if you're reading this to better understand women, you might want to hold the vodka.

Women also worry more about their health, which, ironically, is one of the major factors associated with longevity. The "don't worry, be happy" people—more often men drinking at bars or four-wheeling in the desert—are more likely to die earlier from accidents or preventable illnesses, such as alcoholism, diabetes, hypertension, and heart disease. Those who are appropriately concerned about their health ultimately take better care of themselves and live longer, healthier, and happier lives.

Maybe we should change the phrase from "Don't worry, be happy" to "Be concerned, live longer, be happy!"

Women also engage in fewer behaviors that damage the "executive control center" in the front part of their brains, where decisions are made, self-control is exerted, and forward thinking takes place. Girls are less likely to engage in brain-damaging behaviors such as hitting soccer balls with their heads, or playing tackle football . . . at least they used to be, until the explosion of soccer among young girls.

Women may also live longer than men because they exhibit greater empathy and ability to forgive, which helps them do a better job at weathering the inevitable storms of injustice that rain on us all.

In our own patient outcome studies at the Amen Clinics, both men and women get better at very high rates. Yet our female patients tend to do better, because they are more compliant and take our treatment recommendations more seriously.

Empathic, concerned women aren't just thinking of themselves. They're also thinking about their husbands, which may very well be one reason why married men live longer than unmarried men. I often hear wives nagging their husbands to take better care of themselves. They set out their fish oil capsules and vitamins and encourage them to go to the doctor. Yet, in some studies, married women do not live longer than unmarried women, and they may even have shorter lives. I think the stress of taking care of stubbornly resistant males can wear them out. Here's an example:

Nabil and his wife, Monica, were both physicians who worked to-gether. One day Nabil called his wife saying he vomited and had a bad headache and was not coming to work. Alarmed, Monica told Nabil to go to the hospital. Nabil said he would be okay and that he just needed a nap and hung up the phone. Knowing the symptoms could be serious, Monica called Nabil back and pleaded with him to seek immediate help. Nabil again told his wife he would be ok and not to worry about him. Knowing how much more significant the symptoms could be for people in their early sixties, Monica's worry skyrocketed. She raced home and took Nabil to the emergency room where it was discovered that he had a brain aneurysm. Without immediate medical help, the neurosurgeon told the couple, Nabil would have been dead within an hour.

Women often become the health monitors in their families because they tend to realize and admit problems faster than men. They typically reach out for help and community support years or even decades before their male counterparts. At the Amen Clinics, we see that when a couple is struggling in their relationship, the woman is most often the one who calls for help. Eight out of ten times, when a child is having problems, the mother is the one who calls us, even when both parents work full-time.

Everywhere I look, I see women acting as the health leaders in their families and communities. As one of the cocreators of the Daniel Plan—Pastor Rick Warren and Saddleback Church's program to get the world healthy through religious organizations—I have seen, not surprisingly, that 85 percent of the people who signed up to get healthy in their churches were women.

As a male psychiatrist and physician, I'm increasingly troubled about the way such large numbers of men are falling behind. I remember the day I read that statistic from our research team at Saddleback Church—and had an absolute tantrum! Men have to do better, but it is often at the insistence of our mothers and wives.

In my experience, women are most often the ones who pull the lever for change. They're typically the ones who plan the meals, and they are often the ones who coordinate household activities and oversee the children. Growing up with a powerful matriarch, I learned first-hand that when Mom gets health right, everybody else has the best opportunity to get it right too. And when Mom *doesn't* get it right, that can have a truly devastating effect on both the physical and mental health of the whole family.

During my psychiatric residency training, I studied children and grandchildren of alcoholics. One of my best friends grew up in a severely abusive alcoholic home. One of my research findings was that if your father was an alcoholic it had a significant negative effect on your emotional development. But if your mother was the alcoholic, the devastating effects were much more profound. It is essential to keep the female brain healthy.

Most of this book is devoted to helping you unleash the power of your own female brain. Once you fall in love with your brain and learn how to take care of it, and do the steps I recommend, you'll be able to influence your loved ones and create a brain-healthy community around you, further supporting your own efforts to be well.

In my last book, *Use Your Brain to Change Your Age,* I wrote about Marianne, the western regional director for Franklin Covey, the highly successful training and consulting company. At fifty-nine years old, she felt that her mind was beginning to deteriorate. Physically, she hurt all over and her head felt foggy most of the day. At first she thought that she was just getting older, that she was experiencing something that eventually happens to everyone. But as she got worse, she thought it was unfair to her co-workers that she wasn't at the top of her game, and she considered resigning. She believed her best days were behind her. Then, fortuitously, one of her daughters gave her a copy of one of my programs, which she immediately started. To her amazement, within two months she felt much better. Her pain was gone and the brain fog had lifted. And by staying on the program, within a year she had lost 60 pounds, and her brain felt younger, sharper, and more energized than it had in decades. "I have a fast-acting brain with the wisdom of experience," she told me. "I feel like I am at the peak of my life and my best is no longer behind me."

Recently, Marianne and I were together at a Franklin Covey conference where I was speaking. She told me that as she had gotten healthier one of her daughters got healthier as well. Her daughter had been 140 pounds overweight. But seeing her mother's remarkable progress she wanted the same health benefits for herself and over the next two years lost the 140 pounds. Marianne's remarkable change also inspired her husband to get healthy. In fact, everything at her workplace changed as well. She changed the food at work and was amazed at how much more energy her team had and how much more they accomplished during meetings. "We used to be worn out toward the end of the day. But since we started serving *only* brain-healthy food at work, everyone's energy is up and we are much more productive."

Marianne is the poster female for change in her family, in her business, and her community. My hope is that you will be like Marianne and change your world too.

YET THERE IS EVIDENCE THAT THE FEMALE BRAIN MAY BE IN TROUBLE

According to a recent study, women's life spans in the United States are improving at a slower pace than men's and are actually shorter in many areas than they were two decades ago! Even though women are still expected to outlive men, the study from the University of Washington is cause for concern. The study is based on mortality data by age, sex, and county from 1989 to 2009. In this study, life expectancy for men improved by an average of 4.6 years, but only by 2.7 years for women. The director of the research team expressed his concern, "A gain in life expectancy should be equal among men and women. This is a wake-up call for all of us. It's tragic that in a country as wealthy as the United States, and with all the medical expertise we have, *so many girls will live shorter lives than their mothers*."

Life expectancy stopped improving, or even shortened for women since 1999 in 661 U.S. counties and in 166 counties for men. These declining rates also appear in 84 percent of Oklahoma counties, 58 percent of Tennessee counties, and 33 percent of Georgia counties. According to the research, a larger percentage of women than men are not adequately treating high blood pressure and high cholesterol. Researchers reported that many physicians do not treat women with heart risk factors as aggressively as they do men. Preventable causes, such as tobacco, alcohol, and obesity seem to be at the heart of the lower life expectancies for women.

Across the United States, there is nearly a twelve-year gap in women's life spans. Women live the longest in Collier, Florida (85.8), but have the shortest life spans in McDowell, West Virginia (74.1). In 1989, the gap was only 8.7 years. In Australia, life expectancy improved twelve years in both men and women from 1989 to 2009. We can do better. We can improve longevity if you and your family and friends follow the program in this book.

THE FEMALE BRAIN UNLEASHED

In my family, community, and medical practice, I have seen over and over the amazing change that can result when women understand and take steps to optimize their unique strengths and response to challenges. I have also seen the negative outcomes, including depression, anxiety, and eating disorders, that can result when women do *not* understand their own brains or take the necessary steps to take care of them. In this book I show you, step-by-step, exactly how to unleash the power of the female brain. You'll learn:

- How to fall in love with your brain, so that caring for it becomes a joy and not a burden. It becomes something you *have* to do and a habit you'll love having. It is the expression of a logical mind and self-love.
- How to harness the unique strengths of the female brain, such as empathy, intuition, collaboration, self-control, and a little worry, and how to overcome some of its special vulnerabilities, such as depression, perfectionism, and an inability to let go of negative thoughts
- How to naturally balance the hormones that govern energy, mood, relaxation, power, trust, and lust, and how to make your hormones work for you, instead of against you. You will also learn how to successfully navigate such hormone-related issues as thyroid imbalance, premenstrual syndrome (PMS), polycystic ovary syndrome, perimenopause, and menopause.
- About the different brain types, find out which brain type is yours, and how to use the Amen Clinics Method to optimize your brain
- How to soothe your brain with natural treatments in order to successfully tackle anxiety, worry, depression, perfectionism, and eating disorders. You'll also learn how to turn your brain off, so you're not always bombarded by thoughts of what you have to do next, what might go wrong, or what you fear might be wrong with you.
- How to feed your female brain so that you can flatten your tummy, permanently lose unwanted pounds, get healthy and fit, and stop feeding irritable bowel syndrome, depression, Alzheimer's, and even cancer
- How to get your cravings under control, and boost your decision-making skills to improve your health and weight

- About attention-deficit disorder (ADD) in women, and how, if you have it, it can be sabotaging your success
- About the connection between brain health and beauty, and how taking care of your brain can help you look more vital and younger
- How to optimize your brain for love, sex, and intimacy in relationships. All of these are better when your brain is better!
- How to get your brain ready for babies, raise them in a brain-healthy way, and unleash the power of your daughters' brains
- How to create a brain-healthy community and how doing so can change your world

As a psychiatrist, brain imaging researcher, husband, father of three girls, and brother to five sisters, *I know that women have a unique capability to optimize the potential of their brain,* and I will share the stories of many women, some just like you, who have. Once you unleash the power of your female brain, you can be healthier, live longer, and slow or even reverse the aging process. You can also discover unsuspected reserves of serenity, power, vitality, and love.

DO YOU HAVE TWELVE HOURS TO CHANGE YOUR LIFE?

Everywhere I go people tell me how my work on revitalizing brain health has changed their lives. I know the extraordinary power that can be unleashed when you fall in love with your brain and start loving it and treating it right. I want that success for you, and I know you can have it if you do the right things. To facilitate your success, I will give you twelve simple one-hour exercises to put these brain-healthy principles into your life. These exercises will radically change your life if you do them just as they are outlined. You will see the difference and feel it in your mood, energy, weight, appearance, and mental abilities. Rather than continuing to make decisions that undermine your health, you will know the joy of making great decisions that support your brain and your life. You will experience the benefit of thinking clearly and acting powerfully in a way that follows from healthy, disciplined thought patterns. You will feel the freedom from cravings, worry, depression, and perfectionism, opening up whole new possibilities for every aspect of your life.

Can you get all of this in twelve hours? Yes, you absolutely can.

And then . . . it's up to you. Do you want to keep going in this new, positive direction, falling a little bit more in love with your brain each day? Do you want to keep losing weight, looking great, feeling energized, thinking clearly, acting powerfully? Do you want your life to keep getting better? You *are* on your way. Just keep implementing these twelve simple principles . . . over and over and over. The program will keep getting easier, your life will keep getting better, and you will finally be unleashing the full power of *your* extraordinary female brain.

1

FALL IN LOVE WITH
YOUR FEMALE BRAIN

CARE ABOUT YOUR BRAIN MORE
THAN ANY OTHER BODY PART

*Brain envy is the first step to unleashing the power of the female brain.
My best men are women.*

—WILLIAM BOOTH, THE FOUNDER OF THE SALVATION ARMY
(OVERHEARD COMMENT)

Susan was a forty-five-year-old mother of four and the CEO of a nonprofit company that created educational materials for learning-disabled children. She loved her husband and her family, and she had a strong sense of mission for her work. She was active in her local church and was a respected member of her community. Viewed from the outside, Susan seemed to "have it all."

But when Susan came into my office, she told a very different story. "I'm just not feeling good," she said. "I'm tired all the time, whether I sleep in on the weekends or not! I can't remember the simplest things, and it seems like I can't keep my mind on anything for more than a minute before something distracts me. I am feeling very overwhelmed." She sighed. "And it's getting worse. Stuff I used to be able to do easily I now really have to struggle through. I know people say they slow down as they get older, but I never thought it would happen to me at this age! I wonder if I have early symptoms of Alzheimer's disease. I picked up one of your books and you had such a positive message, that even when we get older, we don't have to *feel* old. That's what I want! But all sorts of things in my body seem to be breaking down. I'm gaining weight. My skin is breaking out—that *never* used to happen! And my cycles feel more jagged and intense. But the worst of it is how crabby and short-tempered I am. My husband keeps telling me I'm always snapping at the children, and at him, and sometimes I don't even realize it!"

THE STRENGTHS AND CHALLENGES
OF THE FEMALE BRAIN

Susan is like so many women I see. She thought she ate a healthy diet but started most days with coffee and a bagel and had a terrible sweet tooth throughout the day. She wanted to work out but could not find the time and consistently drank two glasses of wine at night to relax. There was one major part of her body that she never gave any thought to—her brain. This is ironic, because it is Susan's brain that governs every aspect of her life. Her brain decides what she eats and how much she sleeps. Her brain decides whether to snap at her children or to take a deep breath and try a different approach. And her brain decides whether Susan is going to live a long and vital life looking and feeling her best or whether she is going to age rapidly, look years older than she is, and perhaps even face a serious disorder like cancer, diabetes, heart disease, or Alzheimer's.

Of course, none of these decisions were necessarily conscious. But they were made by Susan's brain nonetheless. And if Susan knew how to take care of her brain, how to give it the biological, psychological, social, and spiritual care it required, then she would be more likely to have a healthy, beautiful brain, which, in turn, would help Susan feel terrific and have the energy she needed to enjoy and be effective in her life.

Brain health is crucial for all my patients: men, women, and children alike. But I have noticed, over many years of practice, that my female patients face special challenges. As we will see in chapter 2, women's brains have five special strengths: empathy, intuition, self-control, collaboration, and a little worry. Empathy allows women to be loving and nurturing. Intuition enables them to quickly grasp information that may not be obvious or easy to justify through logic. Self-control gives them better control over their impulses. Their collaborative gifts help them to work with others. And their tendency to worry, when it's in the right proportions, keeps them focused on possible problems and alert to potential solutions.

So far, so good. But like all gifts, these have their dark sides. Empathy can morph into an overwhelming sense of the world riding on your shoulders, the feeling that you have to take care of everyone before your own needs ever get met. Intuition can awaken anxiety-provoking fears as you "know" something is not right without making sure to check it out or get more information. The brain frequently can misperceive things. Self-control can turn into trying to overcontrol others. Being collaborative can all too easily turn into the feeling that you aren't allowed to do anything until you've gotten agreement from everyone else, such as your co-workers, family, or spouse. And the worry that is so useful in small doses can stress you to the point where it hurts your brain and your body and won't allow you to rest.

Susan too struggled with both the strengths and the challenges of the female brain. Like many women, she felt guilty no matter what she did. If she was home, she was thinking about work; if she was at work, she was thinking about home. A deeply empathetic and caring person, Susan took on everybody's problems as if they were her own. She worried about her personal assistant, who was caring for an elderly mother; her husband, who had come back from the doctor with high blood sugar; and her children, one of whom had just started to date. Susan worried about the learning-disabled students for whom her company produced educational materials. And she worried about her own parents; her mother seemed more forgetful and her father less engaged. Wherever she looked, Susan felt as though there was another demand she should be meeting, another problem she should be solving, another person to whom she could be giving just a little bit more. She just felt as though whatever she did, she could never win. So of course when her husband approached her for sex or even for an affectionate night of cuddling in front of the TV, Susan couldn't stay in the moment and enjoy their time together. She just couldn't turn off her busy brain.

"Susan," I said to her after hearing about her concerns, "it sounds like you are taking care of everyone in your life. But it is time to start taking much better care of yourself. Everyone you care about will be better if you are at your best."

Susan looked at me and asked, "How do I start?"

WHY YOUR BRAIN MATTERS!

Your Brain Is Involved in Everything You Do

It makes the healthy choices or the unhealthy choices that make you feel good or bad.

When Your Brain Works Right, *You* Work Right

Your reactions and decisions benefit you.

When Your Brain Is Troubled, *You* Have Trouble in Your Life

Your bad choices complicate everything.

You Can Change Your Brain and Enhance Your Life!

Following brain-healthy guidelines can give you a fresh start.

THE FOUR CIRCLES APPROACH TO YOUR FEMALE BRAIN

At the Amen Clinics, we have developed our "Four Circles Approach," which is a "brain smart" comprehensive approach to evaluating and treating our patients. You are always more than your symptoms, and to be well it is critical to take into account all aspects of your biology, psychology, social connections, and spiritual health. Our success rates with patients are very high because we take an integrated approach to understanding and healing the brain. If any one of these areas is not optimized, your brain will suffer, and so will your health, well-being, appearance, mood, and relationships.

With Susan, I went to the whiteboard in my office and drew four big circles. In the first circle I wrote *Biology* and began with a set of questions to look at the biological factors influencing her brain. I discovered that no one in her extended family had a history of Alzheimer's disease or other dementia-like processes, but there was a family history of depression. Susan wasn't on any medications. Her diet was not great, which, as we'll see in chapter 5, is a terrible thing to do to your brain. She also tended to eat a lot on the run, because she was so busy—also not good for the brain.

Another big biological problem in Susan's profile was the five or fewer hours of sleep she got each night. I understood her dilemma. With four children and a high-powered job, it was hard to get everything done in a day. But not getting enough sleep is one of the worst things you can do for your brain, so this was a big concern.

As you'll learn in chapter 4, hormones play a huge role in your brain's health, and Susan's hormones were not in the best shape. Her lab results showed that her thyroid levels were low, as were the hormones produced by her adrenal glands (cortisol and DHEA, or dehydroepiandrosterone), likely from chronic stress. Susan basically relied on coffee to get herself going during the day. Then she had a couple of glasses of wine each night to help her relax, which didn't help her hormones, blood sugar, weight, sleep, or her brain. Restoring and balancing Susan's hormones was going to be a key aspect of improving her brain's biological health. I was eager to look at her brain scans (I'll tell you more about this soon) to see what was going on.

First, though, I wanted to see what was happening in the other three circles. In the second circle I wrote the word *Psychology*. Psychologically, Susan was thinking in undisciplined and negative ways; her busy brain kept returning to the same worries, anxieties, and self-criticisms: *I should have done that differently. She probably doesn't like me. I'm not doing enough for him. What is wrong with me, anyway?* Like many female brains, Susan's was prone to a kind of perfectionism in which she magnified her flaws and minimized her good points. In Susan's mind, the few extra pounds she had put on felt like the ultimate proof that she was old and ugly. Her children's normal childhood crises were clear evidence of Susan's not being a good enough mother. And her husband's frustration with Susan's short temper seemed like a sign (completely incorrectly, as it turned out) that their marriage was in trouble.

These psychological issues were both the result of Susan's poor brain health and a contributing factor to it. Thinking in undisciplined, negative ways is just not good for the health of your brain, which is why, in Chapter 6, I teach you how not to believe every stupid thought you have. I refer to these "automatic negative thoughts" as ANTs, and I'll show you several simple, effective ways of ridding yourself of them.

In the third circle I wrote *Social Connections*. There too Susan's brain was facing a number of challenges. Susan felt separated from the most important people in her life, distant from her husband and irritable with her kids. At work, she felt overwhelmed. The support she might have gotten from friends or from her community at church seemed out of reach, because Susan felt too exhausted to reach out.

In the last circle I wrote *Spiritual Health*. As it happened, Susan's brain was in good shape in this circle. She had a deep sense of meaning and purpose in her life that sustained her, even in this challenging time. She felt her work mattered to others, and she knew that her presence at home was crucial for her husband and children. She had a deep sense of connection to God, the planet, and the future. Susan's brain definitely benefited from her sense of meaning and purpose.

Having evaluated each of Susan's four circles, I moved on to look at Susan's brain SPECT scans. One of the unique aspects of our work that differentiates us from most psychiatrists is our belief that we should actually look at and evaluate the organ we treat. We do a brain imaging study called SPECT (single photon emission computed tomography) that evaluates brain blood flow and activity patterns. It looks at how the brain works. At the Amen Clinics we have been performing SPECT scans for twenty-two years and have a database of over seventy-eight thousand scans, giving us a significant edge on how to use them. SPECT scans basically show us three things: areas of the brain that work well and display good activity, areas of the brain that are low in activity, and areas of the brain that are high in activity.

Susan's SPECT scans helped me get an even clearer picture of what was going on with her. I could see that she had low activity in her temporal lobes, the memory areas of her brain, which explained her forgetfulness. She also had low activity in an area of her prefrontal cortex (PFC)—the "executive control" center in the front third of her brain, associated with focus, concentration, and impulse control. The low activity in her temporal lobes and PFC are common in low thyroid states. I suspected that these problems would improve significantly as soon as Susan started taking better care of her brain: balancing her hormones, getting the food, supplements, sleep, exercise, and psychological help she needed, as well as getting more social support from her loved ones and her community.

Susan was also experiencing problems in her limbic system, her "emotional brain." There was increased activity there, probably from the chronic stress that she felt at work, at home, and every place else. Driving out the ANTS would help calm this part of Susan's brain, as would meditation, self-hypnosis, and other relaxation techniques. Healthy food, sleep, a multiple vitamin, fish oil, optimizing her vitamin D level, other targeted supplements, and exercise would help too.

I showed Susan her scan and a healthy one for comparison and pointed out each one of the areas that could use help. As soon as Susan saw her scan and understood what it meant, she asked if it could be made better. This is a question I love answering. The last twenty-two years of my life have been focused on changing my patients' brains and changing their lives. "Yes," I said. "If you follow the program I give you, your brain can become much healthier and you will feel much better." That got her excited.

"You're telling me if I do a better job of taking care of my brain, that this isn't permanent, right?" she said to me. "If I do the right things, I could have a better brain."

"That's right," I assured her. "You have to start thinking and caring about your brain."

Healthy Brain SPECT Scans

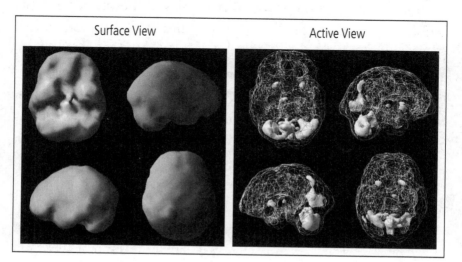

Surface View   Active View

"Starting now," she said, "I want a better brain and a better life." Her face broke out into a smile. "This is just the best news I've heard in a long time," she added. "What do I do? Let's get started."

Susan had just developed brain envy.

Susan's SPECT Scans

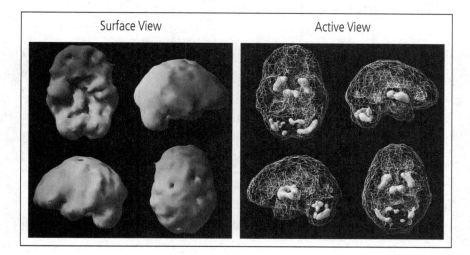

Surface View · Active View

FALLING IN LOVE WITH YOUR BRAIN

What happened to Susan happens for many of our patients who see their brain SPECT scans: They fall in love with their brains. Seeing the images gives them hope and helps them resolve to do things differently. They develop brain envy and want to have a better brain.

Susan began to make changes right away. She told me she would clean up her diet, start getting exercise, make sure to sleep more, and work with me on her thyroid and adrenal gland issues. She learned how to kill the ANTS and set better boundaries with her loved ones so that she wasn't immediately taking everyone else's problems onto her own shoulders.

At the same time, Susan resolved to spend more quality time with her kids—not *more* time but *better* time. As we'll see in chapter 11, mothers often feel so wracked with guilt that they end up doing too much. Then they wear themselves out. I told Susan that good parenting doesn't take an inordinate amount of time; it just takes consistent time. I suggested a powerful exercise you will learn in chapter 11. She agreed, and found that she and her children all got along better as a result.

Susan started playing "Chloe's Game" with herself and her children. This is an exercise I have done with my daughter Chloe since she was two years old. In the game you ask yourself, "Is this good for my brain or bad for it?" I suggested that throughout the day, whatever actions she took, she should ask herself this simple question. The answers helped keep Susan and her children making brain-healthy decisions. I have a close friend in Hong Kong who plays the game with his four-year-old daughter, Kaitlyn. She likes to call it Kaitlyn's Game.

I saw Susan again about a month later, and she was already improving. She had lost 8 pounds and laughed about the time at the gym when her pants were so loose they fell down. "Thank goodness," she said, "it was an all-girls' class." Her skin looked younger, and she was more optimistic. Her energy, mood, and outlook were better too.

I love success stories! What is truly wonderful about Susan's story is that it can be yours too. But the first step is falling in love with your brain, a radical new concept.

THE NEED FOR BRAIN ENVY

Your brain is involved in everything you do. It is your brain that decides when you get married and when you get divorced. It is your brain that manages your money and helps you be successful at work. And it is your brain that determines how healthy you are and whether or not your cravings are under control. When your brain works right, you work right. When your brain is troubled you are much more likely to have trouble in your life. Yet most women never really think about their brains, which is a huge mistake, because success in everything you do starts with a healthy brain.

You don't think about your brain because you cannot see it.

You worry about the wrinkles in your skin because you can see them. You fret about your waistline because zipping up your jeans is taking more and more effort. And you become concerned about the gray in your hair and make an appointment with the hairdresser because your roots stare back at you in the mirror. Your body gives you feedback when it is not doing well. Your brain, on the other hand, only gives you an indirect glimpse that something is not right when your mood is off, you can't sleep, or you start dropping words that used to roll off your tongue.

I never really cared much about my own brain until I started my brain imaging clinical work. I had no problem doing jumps on my bicycle and falling on my head when I was ten. That's what tough boys did. I just got back up. I had no problems playing tackle football and using my helmet to make tackles. The helmet made me feel invincible. I never gave one thought to the first bout of viral meningitis (a brain infection) I had in basic training when I was in the U.S. Army or to the second bout I had during my medical internship. I didn't see any problem with drinking a half gallon of soda a day, carrying around extra weight, or being constantly stressed in medical school and beyond. I was tough! Even as I progressed through my psychiatric training and starting a private practice, I never really thought about my brain. If a physician who specializes in diseases of the brain doesn't really think about his brain, why would you?

It all changed in the spring of 1991. At the time I was the director of a dual diagnosis unit in a northern California hospital, taking care of substance abusers who also had psychiatric issues, and running a very busy practice. Every week, the hospital physicians met for "grand rounds," our weekly educational conference. One day, Dr. Jack Paldi, the chief of medicine at a local general hospital, gave a talk on the practical application of a new brain imaging technology called SPECT, which is a nuclear medicine study that looks at blood flow and activity patterns in the brain. CAT scans and MRIs look at the brain's anatomy; SPECT looks at how the brain functions. Dr. Paldi said that SPECT and studies like it would revolutionize psychiatry. Instead of using educated guesswork to help patients, we would finally have more useful information on the organ we were actually treating, the brain. He showed us SPECT scans of normal people and compared them to the scans of people with Alzheimer's disease, strokes, brain trauma, and seizures.

I was riveted. I had waited a long time for this day in psychiatry. We were the only medical specialty that never looked at the organ we treated, and so I often felt in the dark with my patients. I felt that I needed more information to help me understand their brains so I could better target what I did for them. That lecture changed the trajectory of my personal and professional life.

Over the course of the next few months, I ordered many SPECT scans on my patients and found them extremely useful. They were so valuable that I also started scanning people in my own family: my aunt who had a panic disorder, a cousin who was suicidal and depressed, my children, and then myself. Like many men, I had the belief that I was 100 percent normal, maybe even a little better than normal. Despite my history of playing football and meningitis, I expected to see a very healthy brain. After all, I had never done any illegal drugs, didn't smoke, and rarely drank alcohol.

And yet my brain did not look healthy. In fact, it looked older than I was. It actually had a toxic look.

"Yuck," I thought. "I need to do better."

That same week I also scanned my sixty-year-old mother, Dorie, who had an unbelievably beautiful brain. In fact, she later became our poster example of a healthy brain. Her brain was full, even, symmetrical, and showed healthy activity throughout. Her great brain function was reflected in the myriad healthy activities and relationships she had. She has always been the best friend to her seven kids, twenty-two grandkids, and ten great-grandkids. I had brain envy. I wanted my brain to be like hers.

From that moment on, I have thought about ways to optimize my brain and the brains of my patients, readers, family, and friends. Working to improve my own brain function eventually led me to have a better body. With better function in the front part of my brain that houses judgment and impulse control, my decisions were better, as were my forward-thinking skills.

Brain envy made my life better and I want the same for you.

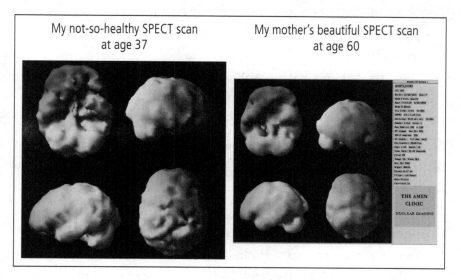

My not-so-healthy SPECT scan at age 37

My mother's beautiful SPECT scan at age 60

It is clear that our society is going the wrong way in terms of female brain health.

Most people just don't care about their brains. We let our little girls hit soccer balls with their heads, do dangerous gymnastic routines, and be flyers in cheerleading, where they are much more vulnerable to brain injuries. There is little brain envy because most people never look at or think about their brains. Since most people never get their brains scanned or tested they have no idea when it starts to look troubled.

When our patients see their own brain scans, they often develop brain envy and want their brain to be better. I once treated a nineteen-year-old woman who was a frequent cocaine abuser. But when she saw on the scan what the cocaine was doing to her brain, she immediately stopped! She was a very smart young lady, and as she looked at the scan, she said, "Uh-oh, my brain runs my life and it's not doing a good job because I am hurting it!" And when I told her that her brain would not finish developing until she was twenty-five and that her drug abuse might permanently delay her development, she said, "Oh, I don't want that!" and just stopped using altogether. I was so proud of her, and I was even prouder when years later she became a health care provider.

I also treated an amazing woman whose mother and grandmother both had died with Alzheimer's. In her family, the women had a higher incidence of Alzheimer's, and this woman wanted to know her own vulnerability. When she got scanned, she saw the developing tendency and realized she was in trouble. As a result, she totally shifted everything in her life—diet, exercise, sleep, and stress—to take better care of herself. Today, she is in her late seventies and is still mentally alert, sharp, and clear-headed. I am very proud of her too.

Women face some special challenges, but they also enjoy unique strengths, one of which is admitting the need for help and seeking it when needed. If you are not taking good care of your brain, you are probably going to face some big problems, either coming up soon or looming down the road. But the good news is that if you develop brain envy, fall in love with your brain, and take better care of it, you can turn everything around.

BOOSTING YOUR BRAIN'S RESERVE IS CRITICAL

One of the most important discoveries I have made through our brain imaging work is a concept I call brain reserve, which is the extra cushion of healthy brain function you have to deal with when stresses come your way. The more brain reserve you have, the better you can cope with the ups and downs of your life. The less brain reserve you have, the harder it is for you to handle stress, hormonal swings, aging, and injuries. Without sufficient brain reserve, you are far more likely to gobble up a bag of Oreo cookies or down multiple glasses of wine as a coping mechanism. So developing as much brain reserve as possible is essential, and the program in this book will help you do just that.

Brain reserve is not a static resource but one that changes constantly, depending on the challenges we face and the care we take of ourselves. From the moment we are conceived, if the environment is healthy, our brain develops with a great deal of reserve to handle the regular stresses of life. If your mother was healthy when she was pregnant with you, took her vitamins, lived in a clean environment, and was not under inordinate stress, you likely were born with a great deal of reserve. If, however, she didn't want you, was chronically stressed, didn't sleep, drank alcohol, smoked, used drugs, had poor nutrition, or was exposed to environmental toxins, such as mercury, lead, mold, or synthetic chemicals, then you were born with less reserve and resilience.

In the same way, the rest of your life either enhances or depletes your reserve. If as a child you were nurtured, mentally stimulated, nourished, and kept safe in a clean environment, your brain had the chance to build and strengthen its reserve. But if you were abused, neglected, or fed junk food, or if you played contact sports, had mono, or were chronically stressed, then your brain reserve was diminished.

Again, as a teen and young adult, being well nourished and living in a stimulating, healthy, socially connected environment continues to build your reserve. But if you smoked pot, drank alcohol, ate poorly, were sleep-deprived, had a concussion, and/or suffered from mood swings or isolation, your reserve was continually being eroded.

Throughout our lives, we are either building or stealing from our brain's reserve. When women or men become symptomatic, such as when you struggle with your mood, memory, or brain fog, it means your brain's reserve has been depleted. Many people erroneously believe that as we age, memory problems, depression, and brain fog are normal. They are not. They are a sign your brain's reserve has been depleted.

You always want to protect your brain's reserve. You do this by first developing brain envy: by caring about your brain. Then you need to avoid anything that hurts it while you engage in regular brain-healthy habits. By the end of this book, it will be crystal clear how to take good care of your brain. But first, you have to care. This is why I want you to develop brain envy. It will keep you motivated to protect your brain's reserve.

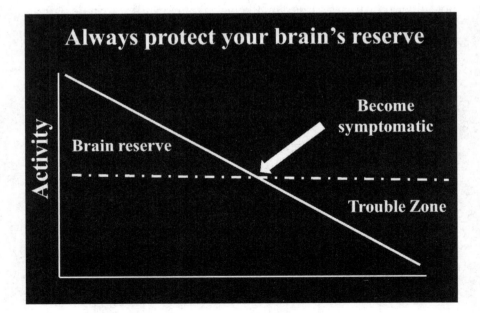

PROTECT YOUR BRAIN'S RESERVE

Think about your family, friends, and co-workers. When there's a crisis, do some of them completely fall apart—racing for the candy bowl, reaching for a pack of cigarettes, or searching for solace in drugs and alcohol—while others manage to maintain their lives in a healthy way? Have you ever wondered why that is? I have. In my work, I have noticed that stressful events, such as the loss of a loved one, being laid off from work, or going through a divorce, can lead to depression, changes in weight, a lack of motivation to exercise, and bad daily habits in some people but not in others. Part of this difference is caused by the level of brain reserve each person has developed over the years.

Boosting brain reserve may even be more important for the female brain, because according to some studies, women are more prone than men to dementia illnesses, such as Alzheimer's.

I remember my patient Kimiko, a lovely young Japanese woman who struggled with learning problems. As a result, she had always felt stupid, especially because in her culture, education was considered critical and there was a lot of pressure to perform. Under the circumstances, Kimiko had really come to hate herself.

Her brain SPECT scan showed overall low activity. I discovered that her APGAR scores, measurements of the health of a newborn in terms of appearance, pulse, grimace, activity, and respiration, were very low, indicating that she likely had oxygen deprivation at birth. When I shared that information with Kimiko, she was so overcome that she couldn't speak for a while. Then she said, so quietly I could barely hear her, "The problem is not me. It is something that happened to me." The scans had actually helped wash away her shame!

A moment later, Kimiko asked me, "Can we make it better?" And as I explained to her the brain-healing steps she could take, the approach that you will learn throughout this book, I could see her excitement begin to grow. Her anxiety turned into enthusiasm and her self-loathing gave way to an open spirit. You can see her before and after scans below.

Kimiko's Scans Before and After Treatment

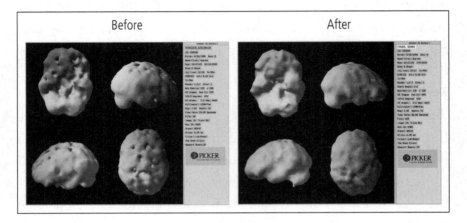

Before   After

HOW BRAIN HEALTH CHANGES EVERYTHING
FOR YOU AND THOSE YOU LOVE

Falling in love with your brain won't just change your life. It can completely transform the lives of everyone you love. Just consider the story of Fatima, who worked with me on an important project to bring my work into corporations around the world.

At the time, she was repeatedly encouraging her husband to get healthy, but like many husbands, Rob was not paying attention. He was forty-four and had back problems, arthritis in his knees, insomnia, and a sluggish memory. After knee surgery, his doctor told him that he would never run again. His father had his first heart attack at age forty and died at fifty-eight. Fatima was concerned. In addition, their boys, ages ten and thirteen, were both struggling in school. As Fatima watched the DVDs of my program, Rob and the boys decided to join her. As they watched the shows, brain envy started to take over in their household and everything in their family has changed, from their diet, to their activity level, to making smarter choices.

From Fatima:

After watching your program, we all fell in love with our brains, especially Rob. He began following your brain-healthy nutrition plan and has lost 39 pounds in just a few short months. He feels great! He gave up virtually all refined sugar, all juices and sweet drinks, drastically cut dairy and gluten, and has dramatically increased his vegetable intake. He also began taking fish oil, vitamin D, a high-quality multivitamin every day and supplements for his brain and says his memory, brain function in general, creativity, and mood have all been boosted. He is also sleeping much better and doesn't get restless leg syndrome anymore. Rob says that he really resonates with the way you explain brain health. He says you are very logical and easy to understand, and because of you he has become much more "thoughtful" in his diet choices, seeing each choice of a "best value" for spending his calories. Rob's pain is gone and he has just finished his second triathlon this year, both times coming in first for his age group. At work, in a meeting recently he was able to come up with the name of a client they had seen twelve years earlier.

Kaden, age thirteen, was struggling in school, mostly C's, a couple of D's which is alarming because he is really bright. All his teachers said although he was a polite kid, he was having trouble focusing and staying on task, and frequently "spaced" homework assignments. At home, Kaden was argumentative, complained about not being able to focus on homework, and had begun looking for disagreements with his little brother which was out of character for Kaden.

Sage, age ten, was a little crankier than usual and grades were A's and B's, although he is capable of straight-A work. His teachers said he was rushing through school assignments and not checking his work.

We followed your recommendations for each and limited TV and video games to no more than a combined total of a half hour per day. We upped their exercise opportunities and put them on fish oil, a high-quality multi, and L-tyrosine, with a high-protein breakfast and regular protein snacks throughout the day.

When we went to parent–teacher conferences one month later, all seven of Kaden's teachers commented that he had made "dramatic improvement," and some of them said, "Whatever you're doing different, please keep it up." Kaden now has straight A's in all of his classes, is listening really well at home and is getting along much better with his brother.

Sage has straight A's and has been able to slow down and focus more on checking his work. He is much more amiable at home when he doesn't play video games.

Now that Rob had such great improvement, his mom and siblings also got on the program.

Because of the changes in the household, I am less stressed and happier as well. Thanks so much for your life changing insights! Our family has really benefited from your programs!

I share this message because I want you to see the power that women can have to change not only their own brains, but also the brains and bodies of those they love. The contrary is also true: If your brain habits are not healthy, it is less likely that your family's will be.

I don't write this to make anyone feel guilty; so many women just don't know the right things to do. I share these stories to motivate you to change and help me change the world now that you have new information. It is common for women to come up to me and say that they have been doing all the wrong things at home and they are concerned about children who are overweight or struggle with behavioral problems. They feel tremendous guilt and sadness. The bad feelings are not helpful for you unless you use the new information to make a significant change for yourself and those you love.

When you get the message in this book, you, like Fatima, can transform everything in your life, and in the lives of those you love. Mari is another example.

Mari

Mari, forty-four, is an award-winning CEO of a fast-growing sheet metal company. She is a rare woman in a macho, man's business world. Yet her road to the top was not easy and had many horrifying turns along the way.

Mari grew up as a latchkey kid with an unreliable, single mother in an unpredictable, chaotic environment that often left her anxious, stressed, and alone. As a way to show love, her mother fed Mari fast food, candy, or cookies. Perhaps as a way to gain some semblance of control over her life, as a teenager she developed bulimia (a common eating disorder that often includes bingeing on high-carbohydrate foods and purging with self-induced vomiting, laxatives, and excessive exercise). And she smoked marijuana and drank alcohol as a way to soothe herself. Given her upbringing, it was not surprising that her first husband, Joe, a sheet metal contractor, had his own struggles with alcohol and drugs.

After they started having children, Mari's maternal instincts told her that the drugs and alcohol had to stop. "The party's over," she told Joe. But for him it was not that easy. The tension and distance in their marriage escalated and a few years later she asked for a divorce. They tried to patch things up, but it wasn't working, and to her regret Mari found herself involved in an affair.

When Joe found out, his world crashed down around him. He told all of their friends and neighbors that Mari was a whore, including the psychiatrist they saw. She was wracked with guilt and shame. A year later, Joe was taking an antianxiety medication that lowers brain function and an antidepressant that also lowers brain function; all the while, he was still drinking (which also lowers brain function), and he kept getting worse and worse. Mari's intuition was that Joe would either hurt himself or someone else. She told her fear to the psychiatrist at their last appointment. "She didn't listen to me because I was the whore who caused all the misery." A day later, Joe called Mari and pleaded with her to come to his office. But her intuition told her it was dangerous and she didn't go. Later that evening, Joe shot and killed himself. The police later said if she had gone to the office, Joe would have likely killed her too.

Mari's life was a blur for the next few years. Before his death, Joe had stopped paying taxes, and the business was upside down. She had to deal with devastated children, probate, a business that was in trouble, the IRS, and her own guilt. But through the help of her faith and friends, she was able to forgive herself and she started to rebuild the business. She found that she had a knack for it and within three years the business turned a profit. Now her business is thriving and she has more than one hundred employees. In 2011, Mari was given the Orange County Business Journal's Excellence in Entrepreneurship Award and the National Association of Women Business Owners Innovator Award.

Still, however, Mari struggled with bulimia and the feelings of anxiety and insecurity. She learned about my work through her church and then saw my programs on public television. She wanted to be better. One day I got a call from my sister Mary, who was one of Mari's best friends. Mari left Mary a voicemail saying she wanted a better brain. "I totally have 'brain envy' and want to do everything I can to get truly healthy, physically and emotionally, for myself, my children, and my business."

Mari then attended one of the groups at the Amen Clinics taught by my wife, Tana, who showed her how to eat right, exercise, take some simple supplements, and do all the things it would take to have a better brain and a better body. The program also included information on controlling negative thought patterns and behavioral issues. Within a few weeks, Mari said her brain was much sharper and that she was better at work. In fact, during the class her business closed a million-dollar deal, which Mari said was due in part to her better brain function. "If I had not gotten clear-headed, I might have missed the window of making this deal." Since being on our brain-healthy program Mari reports that she is more focused, stays on task better, holds people more accountable at work, is less distracted, and less reactive to her day.

Mari's habits have rubbed off on her children, and she has started to implement changes at work. Mari wants her employees to benefit from the program and has started to take steps to create a brain-healthy company.

Women like Mari can change their brains . . . change their lives . . . change their worlds.

Hour 1 Exercise—Brain Envy: Why Do You Care?

Unleashing the power of the female brain starts with brain envy. You have to want to have a better brain. When I say this in lectures, people laugh. It is such a foreign, funny concept, but since your brain controls everything you do, getting it to function at its best will improve everything in your life from your relationships to work, finances, and physical health.

For you to consistently make the right decisions regarding your brain, you must have a burning desire to get it healthy. Why do you care about your brain? Write it down and look at it every day.

Write down at least five important reasons to get healthy, such as:

- · Living longer
- · Looking younger
- · Feeling happier

- Feeling calmer and more relaxed
- Making better decisions
- Having better energy
- Increasing mental clarity
- Being a better role model for my children
- Having greater self-esteem
- Looking better in jeans or a bathing suit
- Being able to participate in sports and other activities I used to enjoy
- Having a better relationship with my spouse
- Reversing diabetes, heart disease, or other health risks
- Decreasing my risk for Alzheimer's disease and other diseases of aging
- Having the confidence to apply for the job I really want

1. _____

2. _____

3. _____

4. _____

5. _____

Once you write these down, post them where you can see them every day. Knowing your motivation is essential to wanting to do the right things for your brain.

ANCHOR IMAGES

Fifty percent of the brain is dedicated to vision. Having visual cues and reminders about brain envy is a very effective tool to help you stay on track. For me, I have pictures that remind me why I need and want a great brain. I have pictures of my wife, four children, and five grandchildren everywhere. Plus I have special "anchor" images that remind me in an instant why I want a better brain.

As I write this, one of my grandchildren is sick. Emmy has a very rare genetic deletion syndrome, which causes bad seizures and developmental delay. In the first month of her seizures, in one day, she had 160 seizures. I need to be here and be healthy to help Emmy and my daughter Breanne for as long as I can. If I am not healthy, I will never be my best for the people who need me. I never want to be a burden to my children. I want to be the leader of my family, but the only way that is possible is if I have a good brain. I post my anchor images where I can see them every day, to remind me why I need to stay healthy. I suggest you do the same.

My Anchor Images of Emmy

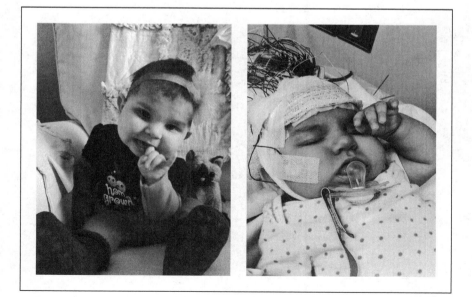

THE FORK-IN-THE-ROAD EXERCISE

One of my favorite exercises with my patients is one I call the Fork in the Road. Here I want you to vividly imagine a fork in the road with two paths.

To the left, imagine a future of pain. If you don't care about your brain and just keep doing what you've always done, what will your life be like in a year? In five years? In ten years? I want you to imagine your brain continuing to get old and all that goes with that: brain fog, tiredness, depression, memory loss, and physical illness.

To the right, imagine a future of health. If you care about your brain and do the exercises I recommend, what will your life be like in a few days, in a year? In five years? In ten years? I want you to imagine your brain getting healthier and younger and all that goes with that: mental clarity, better energy, a brighter mood, great memory, a trimmer, healthier body, healthier skin, and a younger brain.

2

HARNESS THE UNIQUE STRENGTHS
OF THE FEMALE BRAIN

USE YOUR INTUITION, EMPATHY,
COLLABORATION, SELF-CONTROL,
AND A LITTLE WORRY TO GIVE YOURSELF
A GREAT ADVANTAGE

*Nurturing your strengths and protecting against your vulnerabilities
is the second step to unleashing the power of the female brain.
If you want anything said, ask a man. If you want anything done,
ask a woman.*

—MARGARET THATCHER

M ale and female brains are different. I know some people will be irritated when they read this. They want us all to be the same. But after looking at seventy-eight thousand brain SPECT scans over the last twenty-two years, it is just so.

In a research project in which we compared fifty healthy, age-matched male and female SPECT scans, the results showed that women had significantly overall increased activity compared to men. In the images below, the shaded color shows the areas of increased activity in the female brain compared to male brains. In our study, we did not find any decreases in activity in women compared to men. This is very consistent with our extensive clinical experience. Women have busy brains; men's are a lot quieter. One pattern is not better than the other; they are just different.

We're not completely different, of course, but we are different in subtle ways that can have a big impact. These differences are often reflected in the way the two genders interact with each other; and maybe why we so often misunderstand each another and can so easily get on each other's nerves.

Blood Flow Differences Between Female and Male Brains

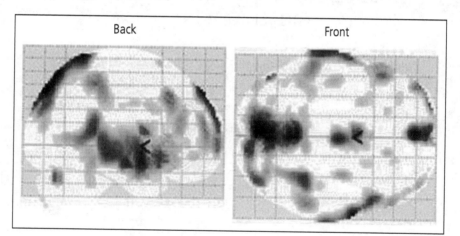

A word of caution: These are measurable differences that always fall within a range of responses with a lot of overlap between groups. Obviously, not all women are the same. Nor are all men the same. Some women have low activity in their brains, some men (me, for example) have high activity. Some women's brains act more like the average man's, and some men's brains act more like the average woman's. There is evidence that the brains of homosexual or bisexual individuals may lie somewhere in between. Both men and women can be great mathematicians, engineers, doctors, lawyers, astronauts, cooks, real estate agents, parents, and caregivers.

But overall, there are significant brain differences between the sexes that can be measured in a laboratory, seen on a brain scan, and observed in our everyday lives. Even when men and women succeed at the same task, they may call on different strengths and areas of the brain to do it.

WHY THE DIFFERENCES?

At the very beginning of life, you can't see any differences between the male and female brain. In fact, in the early stages of development in the womb, male and female fetuses both have female brains. But it doesn't stay that way for long. And it's all because of a Y chromosome.

We're all born with a blueprint that provides the instructions for how we will develop. The individual instructions are in our genes, and the genes are clustered onto chromosomes. A human has twenty-three pairs of chromosomes, with one member of each pair coming from our mother and the other from our father.

The sex of a baby is determined by one particular pair made up of either XX or XY chromosomes. If both chromosomes are of the X variety, the baby will be a girl. If one is an X and the other a Y, the baby will be a boy. Mothers always contribute an X chromosome (that's all they have). Fathers can contribute either an X or a Y chromosome (they have one of each), so it is the father who determines the sex of the baby.

The Y chromosome in the male fetus is very important, because, among other things, it gives the instruction for the male testicles to wake up and start producing large amounts of testosterone halfway through the pregnancy. As a result, between eighteen and twenty-six weeks, an irreversible transformation in structure takes place that stamps the brain as recognizably male.

Meanwhile, the hormone estrogen has been bathing the brain of the unborn female, influencing and feminizing the development of her brain.

The difference is so profound that by twenty-six weeks in utero, researchers can use ultrasound to distinguish between male and female brains.

Psychologist Simon Baron-Cohen has been studying the effects of fetal testosterone on brain and child development. In the late 1990s, he launched the Cambridge Longitudinal Fetal Testosterone (FT) Project, a research program that followed children of mothers who had amniocentesis, a procedure where fluid is taken from the womb sack during pregnancy, to study the long term effects of FT. The study revealed that higher levels of FT are negatively correlated with social and language development.

> *As fetal testosterone went up, eye contact, empathy, and the ability to read what was in someone else's mind went down.*

THE SECOND BURST

Hormones come into play again at puberty, when a second burst of testosterone transforms a boy into a man. Around this time, a girl's brain informs her ovaries to produce greater quantities of estrogen and other female hormones that begin to transform her into a woman. With all these hormones surging through their bodies, the adolescent boy and girl become extremely interested in one another.

As with boys, too much testosterone in females can cause social troubles. When Dr. Baron-Cohen and colleagues gave testosterone to a group of sixteen young women, it led to a significant impairment in empathy, even more so if they had been exposed to higher levels of FT. I'll tell you more about high testosterone levels in women when we discuss polycystic ovary syndrome in chapter 4.

SO MUCH ALIKE . . .

Understanding some basic brain anatomy will help you know your brain and to understand some of its unique differences.

The human brain typically weighs about 3 pounds and is the consistency of soft butter. The most noticeable structure in human brains is the cerebral cortex, the wrinkly mass that sits atop and covers the rest of the brain. The cortex has four main areas or lobes on each side of the brain: frontal, temporal, parietal, and occipital.

The frontal lobes consist of the motor cortex, which is in charge of movement; the premotor cortex, which plans movement; and the PFC, which is considered the executive part of the brain. The PFC is the most evolved part of the human brain: It is the center of focus, forethought, judgment, organization, planning, impulse control, and empathy, and it allows you to learn from the mistakes you make. It makes up 30 percent of the human brain. In contrast, our closest cousin, the chimpanzee,

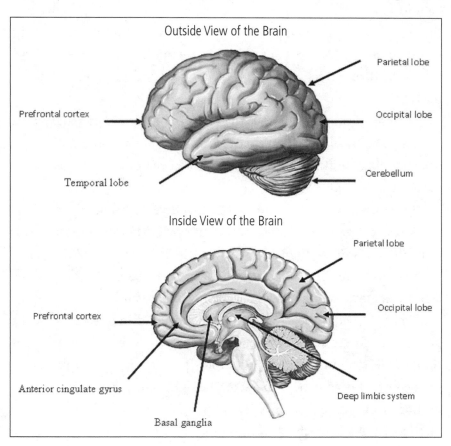

has a PFC that makes up only 11 percent of its brain; a dog's PFC makes up just 7 percent, and a cat, only 3.5 percent. It's a good thing a cat has nine lives, because its PFC isn't going to do much to keep it out of trouble!

As we will see, females typically have a larger PFC, which is associated with increased empathy, focus, impulse control, and self-control.

The temporal lobes, underneath your temples and behind your eyes, are the seat of auditory processing, naming things, getting memories into long-term storage, and emotional reactions. They are the "*what* pathway" in the brain as they name what things are. The parietal lobes, to the top side and back of the brain, are the centers for sensory processing and direction sense. They are the "*where* pathway" because they help us know where things are. And the occipital lobes, at the back of the cortex, are concerned primarily with vision. Information from the world enters the back part of the brain (temporal and parietal lobes), is processed, and then passes to the front part of the brain for decision making.

Sitting beneath the cortex is the deep limbic, or emotional, system. This is the part of the brain that colors our emotions and is involved with bonding, nesting, and emotions. It has been estimated to be larger in women.

The cortex is divided into two hemispheres, left and right. While the two sides overlap in function, the left side in right-handed people is generally the seat of language, which is why it is considered the dominant hemisphere. The left hemisphere tends to be analytical, logical, detail-oriented, and capable of conceiving and executing plans.

The right hemisphere is home to the poet within us. It sees the big picture, the forest to the left hemisphere's trees. It sees patterns and is responsible for hunches and intuition. It allows people to recognize problems that need to be addressed. The right hemisphere features connections from more distant parts of the brain, so it can draw on many different inputs to reach its conclusions.

In his book *The New Executive Brain*, Dr. Elkhonon Goldberg describes that novel activities are processed preferentially in the right hemisphere whereas activities that are more routine become managed by the left hemisphere.

Compared to the left hemisphere, the right hemisphere also tends to be more fearful, anxious, and pessimistic. The right hemisphere develops earlier and more quickly than does the left. This may be why the default human position seems to be negative (lots of ANTs—automatic negative thoughts). When we are young and helpless, we tend to experience the world through the right hemisphere with its negative bent.

Damage to the right hemisphere has been shown to give people a higher level of subjective well-being (by damping down the anxious tendencies), and some of these people may end up in denial about serious problems. I think this is why at the Amen Clinics we tend to see people who have left-sided brain problems more than right-sided trouble.

It's almost as though there are two personalities with the human being, each represented by one of the hemispheres. But fortunately, in healthy brains, the two sides do not work independently. Instead, they work in concert together to make us who we are. This collaboration between the different sides of the brain is made possible by three nerve bundle connections that enable them to share information; the largest of these is the corpus callosum.

EQUALLY SMART, DIFFERENTLY WIRED

The most obvious difference between male and female brains is that the former is larger, about 8 percent to 10 percent on average. That's no surprise, since male bodies are larger overall. However, even correcting for total body weight, it has been estimated that men have 4 percent more neurons or brain cells than women. When I was on Carolyn Davidson's radio show in Dallas, she asked me, "Why do men need 100 extra grams of brain tissue to accomplish the same things as women?" The size difference is not consistent across the entire brain; some parts of the female brain are larger than the corresponding parts of the male, and vice versa.

Dr. Jill Goldstein of Harvard Medical School used MRI scans to compare male and female brains. She found that *compared to men, women have larger volume in the frontal cortices and limbic cortices.* Remember, the frontal cortex is in involved in many of the higher cognitive functions, including language, judgment, planning, impulse control, and conscientiousness, while the limbic cortices are concerned with emotional responses. This might explain why women tend to be less impulsive and more concerned with emotions than are men, as well as why they have "busy" brains that won't stop worrying. It might also explain the source of the female brain's key strengths: intuition, collaboration, self-control, empathy, and a little worry.

Imaging also consistently shows that the hippocampus, one of the major memory centers in the brain, is larger in women than in men. Men, on the other hand, have bigger amygdalas, the part of the brain that processes fear and anger, which may be why men often jump to those emotions in a crisis. Compared to women, men have larger parietal lobes, which are concerned with the perception of space. Women use language (and collaboration) to ask for directions, men use their parietal lobes to find their own way. Men also tend to have larger volume in the hypothalamus, which is concerned with sexual behavior. It's no wonder that men have a greater interest in sex.

Men and women are equally smart, but each sex tends to use different parts of the brain to solve problems or achieve goals. For example, researchers at the Kennedy Krieger Institute found that male and female brains showed different patterns of *lateralization*, which sides of the brain they used, when performing different types of tasks. During a language task, men seemed to rely almost completely on the left "language" side of the brain, showing more activity there. However, during a visual–spatial task, such as constructing something with blocks, men showed activity on both sides of the brain.

Women, by contrast, showed more activity on both sides of the brain during a language task and were more "lateralized" to the right side during the visual–spatial task. This could explain why women are more adept at language (they use both sides of their brain), while men are more adept at judging distances and making a beeline to where they parked the car.

GRAY MATTER, WHITE MATTER: DOES IT REALLY MATTER?

Well, yes, it does. The percentage of gray matter versus white matter is another key difference between male and female brains. Gray matter is composed mainly of brain cell bodies; while white matter is made up of brain cell tracks (think communication cables) that provide the connections between cells. They appear white because they are covered in a fatty substance known as myelin. Myelin, like insulation on copper wires, helps nerve cells work faster and more efficiently.

A consistent finding is that females have a higher percentage of gray matter compared to males, whereas males have a higher percentage of white matter. But these figures are for the entire brain, and the matter—gray or white—is actually more complicated than it first appears. It turns out that in the parts of the brain that are related to intelligence, the proportions are reversed: Men have more gray matter (6.5 times the amount found in women), whereas women have more white matter (10 times the amount found in men). This means men are likely to do more localized processing of information, using only a few key areas to work through a problem or task, while women draw on many areas at the same time.

What does this mean? According to Richard Haier of the University of California, Irvine, "These findings suggest that nature has created two different types of brains designed for equally intelligent behavior." You see, it's the gray matter that "thinks," but it's the white matter that connects different brain areas so that thinking can benefit from a wider range of information and the relationships between them.

Dr. Haier's work also showed gender differences in the areas of the brain most involved with intelligence. In women, 84 percent of the gray-matter regions and 86 percent of the white-matter regions involved in intelligence were located in the frontal lobes, the "executive" part of the brain that governs, among other things, planning, impulse control, empathy, and worry. Men's front lobes held only 45 percent of their gray matter and 0 percent of their white matter. Instead, for men, the areas of the brain most associated with their intelligence were more on the left side of the brain.

INTUITION: WHY WOMEN JUST "KNOW" THINGS

Like all creatures, we have built-in defense mechanisms. We are not the fastest or most ferocious, but we have big brains! And intuition, or knowing something without knowing how you know it, is one of our strongest assets. Without our being aware of where the information came from or the reasoning process behind it, intuition presents a conclusion to the conscious mind. The unique structure and functioning of your female brain may give you an advantage here.

As a woman, you tend to use broader connections in the brain, whereas a man's brain tends to be more localized. The greater density of white matter in the areas of the brain related to intelligence means that you are more likely making more connections between the different parts of your brain. Compared to a man, you dip more into your right side, which is thought to be the seat of the emotional and spiritual worlds—the source of extrasensory wisdom. This allows you to pick up on more cues and connect them without even being aware that you're doing so.

A woman also senses information based on *gut feelings*. She can sense when a friend or co-worker is depressed, a child is feeling overwhelmed, or a meeting is becoming tense. Brain imaging studies show that females have larger areas in the brain dedicated to track gut feelings, specifically areas deep in the frontal lobes called the insula and anterior cingulate gyrus. The female brain is generally quicker at assessing the thoughts of others based on limited information, gut feelings and hunches.

For many people intuition is hard to accept. Skeptics often describe it as emotional, unreasonable, or unscientific. But Einstein knew better. He wrote:

The intuitive mind is a sacred gift and the rational mind is a faithful servant. We have created a society that honors the servant and has forgotten the gift.

Intuition, in combination with a rational mind, allows us to make predictions that will amaze us. "I knew it," we will say later when our intuition bears fruit.

Throughout time and across cultures, humans have believed that women are able to tap into special sources of knowledge that at times seemed uncanny. My mother always seemed to have eyes in the back of her head and knew instinctively when I was not being 100 percent honest.

Scientific research bears out this cultural wisdom, showing that women pick up more on nonverbal cues, which allows them to be more intuitive and empathic. They also have been shown to be better than men at recognizing facial differences and changing vocal intonations. Ruben Gur, Ph.D., a psychologist and neuroscientist at the University of Pennsylvania, reported that "women are faster and more accurate at identifying emotions."

Why would women develop this kind of interconnectedness leading to intuition to a greater extent than men? Researchers have surmised this skill may have developed because of the special conditions women have always faced, particularly their unique tasks in the human family. First, as caretakers of infants, women have always needed special skills to pick up on the needs of others who could not use language to express themselves. An intuitive woman was better able to help her babies survive. At the same time she had to read and properly respond to the messages of more powerful—perhaps dangerous—males. Her intuitive skill was likely necessary for her survival.

Not all researchers have found women more intuitive than men. In one fascinating study, researchers found that men who were paid to pay attention to their intuition actually were able to perform as well as women on intuitive tasks. The problem, of course, is that intuition can happen at any time, not just when someone else is paying us to pay attention to it.

THE DARK SIDE OF INTUITION

Like all gifts, intuition has its downside. Sometimes intuitive women "know" things that simply aren't true. Rather than check out their perceptions in other ways, they cling to their initial beliefs, which can cause serious problems for themselves and their loved ones.

It is likely best to strive to make decisions with both sides of your brain. If you just make decisions with your intuition, you could get hurt! I have seen women who were married to abusive men, wanting to believe the trauma will not happen again, denying their intuition. Once you have an intuitive thought, ask yourself, "What's the evidence for it?"

Women worry more than men, which makes them better at sniffing out potential problems—but this also makes them prey to negative thoughts that simply lie to them. When you let the ANTS become undisciplined, they infest your mind, and become the seeds for anxiety and depression. If you have a feeling about something, check it out.

Lindora's Intuitive Female CEO

My good friend Cynthia Graff is the CEO of Lindora, a highly successful group of weight-loss clinics in Southern California; it is primarily a female organization. Cynthia places high value on intuition, which she believes offers her company a competitive advantage. "If you tap into your intuition," she says, "you can get me the solutions faster than if you have to wade through all the data."

"Of course, it's important to validate women's intuition," Cynthia warns, as sometimes women's intuition can run away with them. A woman might walk by a co-worker and notice that her co-worker's head is down and that she has a grim, preoccupied look on her face. The first woman can all too easily jump to the conclusion that her co-worker is mad at her, an intuitive read that isn't necessarily correct. Perhaps the co-worker is having a bad day, worried about something at home, or just having gas pains! The intuitive woman will suffer needlessly if she "knows" the worst and doesn't bother to check it out.

This is a problem I have certainly run into with the women in my own life. I often have to say to my wife, daughters, and sisters, "*Please* don't read my mind. I have enough trouble reading it myself!"

Intuitions can be affected by a number of different biological factors, such as how much sleep you've gotten, the time of your menstrual cycle, and whether your blood sugar is high or low. Intuition is far more reliable when you're rested, nourished, and relaxed. And you don't always know when hunger, exhaustion, or menstrual issues are distorting your judgment. Get both sides of your brain involved. If you undervalue your intuition, you're depriving yourself of a special gift; but if you overvalue your intuition, you may make important mistakes.

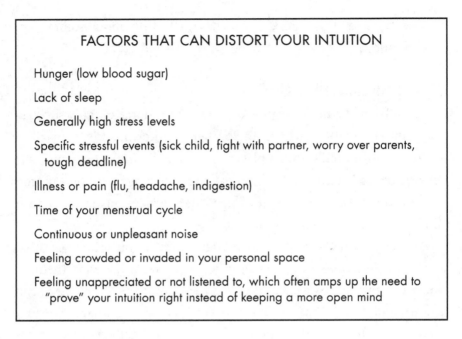

FACTORS THAT CAN DISTORT YOUR INTUITION

Hunger (low blood sugar)

Lack of sleep

Generally high stress levels

Specific stressful events (sick child, fight with partner, worry over parents, tough deadline)

Illness or pain (flu, headache, indigestion)

Time of your menstrual cycle

Continuous or unpleasant noise

Feeling crowded or invaded in your personal space

Feeling unappreciated or not listened to, which often amps up the need to "prove" your intuition right instead of keeping a more open mind

EMPATHY AND COLLABORATION: WHY WOMEN MAY MAKE BETTER BOSSES

Another key strength of the female brain is *empathy,* the ability to recognize and share other people's experiences, to put yourself in another's position and feel what they feel. Within both male and female brains, we have *mirror neurons* that are activated when we empathize or identify with another person. Mirror neurons allow to us actually feel what another person is feeling, which is why we get scared during scary movies and feel sad or even cry during sad scenes. Research demonstrates that women have stronger empathic tendencies than males, which is likely a function of their bulkier frontal lobes. Damage to this part of the brain impairs empathy.

Research published in the journal *Neuroscience* in 2009 reported that females had significantly more gray matter in the regions of the brain's mirror neuron systems compared to males.

WHY WOMEN MAY MAKE BETTER BOSSES

- Increased empathy
- Collaboration
- Concerned about social cohesion of the group
- Less risk-taking behavior
- Bulkier volume in part of the PFC (executive part of the brain), which is the center of judgment, planning, empathy, and impulse control

---

An article in the June 2011 *Harvard Business Review* had an intriguing title: "What Makes a Team Smarter? More Women." The article reported on a study in which teams were given a number of tasks involving brainstorming, decision making, and problem solving. Teams were given collective intelligence scores based on their performance.

Guess which teams did better? If you guessed that it was the teams that had higher individual IQ scores, you would be wrong. The teams that had a higher "group IQ" were the teams with more women.

Why this is so may be found in the work of Simon Baron-Cohen, who identifies two brain types. The male brain relies on systemizing tendencies to figure out how things work. A man searches for the underlying rules governing why a system behaves as it does. The goal is to understand the system so he can predict what will happen next. The female brain is better defined by its empathizing tendencies, which are driven to identify what another is thinking and feeling so that an appropriate response can be made. A woman's goal in this case is to understand another in order to predict behavior and form an appropriate emotional connection.

These differences may appear very early. Dr. Baron-Cohen's research on infants backs previous findings by other researchers that girls are more "people centered." He studied one-day-old infants in the maternity ward by presenting them with either the friendly face of a female student or a mobile that matched the color, size, and shape of the student's face and included a scrambled mix of her facial features. The experimenters, without knowing the sex of the babies, found that the baby girls spent more time looking at the student. The boys spent more time looking at the mechanical mobile. There was a significant difference in social interest of boys and girls, and it was in evidence from the first day of life.

ACCORDING TO SIMON BARON-COHEN'S RESEARCH, HIGHER FETAL TESTOSTERONE IS ASSOCIATED WITH:

- Less eye contact
- Fewer words
- Lower empathy
- Higher tendency to systematize or collect things
- Higher interest in constructing objects
- Lower volume in the planum temporale, the brain area associated with language
- Lower volume in an area of the PFC involved with impulse control

---

Men may be more focused on problem solving, with less concern for the emotional cohesion of a group. They may be less aware of one another and more isolated within themselves. Women tend to be more sensitive to the emotional atmosphere and more inclusive. On the other hand, women can get overemotional and lose their ability to function when negative emotions flare up.

A woman's enhanced empathic response may give her an advantage of building a consensus within a group. Many women leaders encourage collaboration over individual power. And all of this may serve to make her an excellent leader.

Just as women have to be careful with the dark side of intuition, though, they must watch out for the dark side of empathy: codependence or doing too much for others. Another downside is something known as *compassion fatigue*. This is common among therapists and caregivers, who have a much higher percentage of women both professionally (social workers, nurses, home health aides) and personally, such as the mothers of children who are physically disabled, learning-disabled, autistic, or struggling with ADD. After spending hours each day caring for someone in pain, an empathetic person can feel overwhelmed, developing anxiety or depression as a result. It's important to take time to restore yourself so you can continue to care for others and yourself.

Of course, many men are intuitive, compassionate, empathic, and collaborative. It just takes more work and sometimes more incentives for us.

THE STRENGTHS AND CHALLENGES OF A FEMALE WORKPLACE

At Lindora, 99 percent of the staff are female, as are 85 percent of the patients, so Cynthia is quite aware of how the female brain operates in the workplace. I asked her about the strengths and challenges of women in the workplace, and this is how she responded:

> *The culture of our company is very nurturing. We nurture one another so that we can help both our staff and our patients. When I speak about our company culture with some of my fellow male CEOs of health-services companies, they look at me like I am from a different planet. I talked about inspiring the staff to accomplish a goal. They talk about having financial numbers and consequences if people don't produce. I talked about being positive so that negative neurochemical responses don't interfere with productivity. They talked about telling their employees they have to get the job done or they're out of here. They don't understand that if they speak that way to a health care giver, that person is going spend the next couple of hours not able to care for their clients at the same level.*

At Lindora we understand that each person is an essential part of Lindora's success. And that's why each clinic is called a team. We all know that a team is only as strong as the weakest member. One day, I'm strong, another day someone else is strong, and we all try to help one another."

Cynthia explained that the culture in her company is so collaborative and empathic that team members are always checking to see who needs help at the moment. Maybe one day, a particular woman's child is sick, so the others pitch in to cover her workload and cut her some slack. Another day, someone's elderly parent might need extra care, so that is the employee who gets extra support. "Our employees form an informal support network where even without being asked by a direct supervisor, they still volunteer to cover for one another!" she told me. "Men look at our organization, and they can't figure that one out!"

But Cynthia agrees that compassion fatigue is also a challenge. "The nurturing personality type that goes into caregiver professions may have trouble setting boundaries," she says.

Likewise, empathy can be a challenge, as managers don't want to ask their staff to do something that they themselves wouldn't want to do. "As opposed to a top-down directive that says, 'That person is gonna do it, and I don't care what they're thinking about or what implications that's going to have on the rest of their day.' "

Cynthia also views her own success in a collaborative way. "I want to win, but I want that to be by everybody winning," she says. "You get joy by winning—and by helping other people win!"

SELF-CONTROL: LIVING SMARTER, LONGER

Ruben Gur, as others, has found that the PFC, the area of the brain used to control anger and aggression, is larger in females than in males. And research has shown that women are better at keeping strong negative emotions in check. Possibly this is because women's ability to pick up on emotional cues from others gives her the heads-up to diffuse escalating situations. Also, her more empathic brain may respond to others' distress with a wish to calm the situation. To be aggressive would require dampening the more natural empathic response. When she does turn aggressive, she's more likely to produce a verbal attack rather than attack physically. At the end of 2004, of all the prisoners in the United States, only 7 percent were females, indicating females likely have better self-control over their behavior.

In a series of fascinating experiments, Adrienne Raine and colleagues have been looking at brain function in people with antisocial personality disorder (ASD); these are people who chronically break societal rules. Incidence of ASD is much higher in males, as the crime statistics above indicate. When compared to a healthy group, people with ASD had between 9 percent and 18 percent less volume in their PFCs. Women who had antisocial behavior or tendencies also had lower volume in this part of the brain.

A larger PFC may be the secret to a longer, healthier life. Back in the 1920s, American psychologist Lewis Terman initiated a longitudinal study on a large group of 1,548 gifted children. Even though Terman died in 1956, his students at Stanford University, and then their students, continued following up on these subjects as they got older, all the way up until today. And they're still writing about their findings, which give fascinating insight into such questions as what life factors increase success, health, and longevity.

Two of the current researchers, Howard Friedman and Leslie Martin, published an update of results in their recent book, *The Longevity Project: Surprising Discoveries for Health and Long Life from the Landmark Eight-Decade Study*. What was the surprise? It was the conclusion that the secret to living a long life had nothing to do with happiness, a lack of stress, or avoiding hard work. They found that the secret was living conscientiously and using forethought, planning, and perseverance in all aspects of one's life. Conscientiousness was the number-one predictor of longevity.

Friedman offers a number of reasons why conscientious people stay healthier longer and outlive their more frivolous age mates. For one thing, they are less likely to smoke, drink immoderately, abuse drugs, or engage in risky behavior like driving too fast. They are more likely to take their vitamins, wear their seat belts, and follow their doctors' orders. Friedman also suggests that conscientious people are likely to enter into situations and relationships that are healthier. With regard to relationships, the finding is that being loved isn't as important as just having lots of other people in one's life and caring for and helping others. It turns out that it is in fact better to give than to receive.

Having a bigger, stronger PFC helps you live longer, because it is involved in conscientiousness, decision making, and impulse control. Protect your PFC and the quality of your decisions at all costs.

A LITTLE WORRY: A BENEFIT THAT KEEPS HER ON HER TOES

Because of their busier brains, women tend to be worrywarts. They worry over what they eat, how they look, what others think of them, what's going to happen, ad infinitum. It makes sense. Their brains keep talking to them, presenting them with scary scenarios. In our research, we have also seen that an area of the brain called the anterior cingulate cortex is more active in the female brain. This is the part of the brain that helps you shift attention and recognize errors. When it is overactive, people tend to get stuck on negative thoughts or negative behaviors and see what is wrong rather than what is right.

On brain imaging studies, Dr. Mirko Diksic from McGill University found that serotonin production was 52 percent greater in men than in women. Serotonin is one of the most potent calming neurotransmitters in the brain that is involved with mood, sleep, pain, and appetite issues. At the Amen Clinics, we have seen low serotonin levels associated with overactivity on brain SPECT scans in the worry and mood centers of the brain. Given that females tend to have less serotonin than males, it helps to explain why they have a higher incidence of anxiety, depression, and worry. Researchers have shown that women, in fact, respond better to serotonin-boosting medications than men. Much more on this later.

Of course, this doesn't mean that men don't worry or see problems. But men and women tend to worry differently. When women worry, their busy brains and associative thinking powers kick in, which means one worrisome idea quickly connects with others to build momentum that can snowball out of control. A woman is more prone to anxiety so she tends to see negative outcomes in her future rather than positive ones. Her husband's worries are more likely to be confined. He is more likely to compartmentalize his problems.

A woman's brain never seems to rest, not even when she's asleep. For many women, their sleep pattern takes a radical shift after they have their first baby. A woman knows that now she is responsible for someone else, so the typical female brain becomes hyperalert to the responsibility. She must always be concerned for the safety of her infant and herself. This keeps her much more attuned to what's going on around her, taking in information and assessing what it means for the survival of herself and her children.

But a woman need not simply suffer from worry. She can use it to benefit herself and others. Her awareness of problems and her desire to keep her family safe can make her more health conscious. If she channels her worry into action, she's the one who directs the health of her loved ones and makes the home safe. Her worry also gets her to seek help when it's needed. Men are often overly optimistic and may not see a problem that's right in front of them. That's one of the reasons that men don't ask for directions. They don't know they're lost! It's not just a problem when driving. It's a problem in relationships too. Men often simply don't realize there is trouble. Maybe that's why women are more likely to file for divorce or leave a relationship before men.

To admit you're lost, or in a troubled relationship, is to admit a failure, and many men have trouble doing it. To admit you're lost means having to ask for help, and that's something women are good at doing, for themselves and those they care about.

Lower serotonin levels are not all bad. Too much serotonin can be associated with lower motivation and the "don't worry, be happy" syndrome. I have prescribed medications that boost serotonin (selective serotonin reuptake inhibitors, or SSRIs) since 1988 when Prozac was first released onto the U.S. market. One of the first side effects I noticed early on in some people, especially men, was a significant decrease in motivation and the ability to get things done. One business owner told me he felt less anxious, but he was not getting his paperwork done, and that was going to cause real trouble for him at work. Also, on SPECT scans we see that SSRIs lower PFC function and have the potential to disinhibit behavior, sometimes unleashing impulsive sexual or aggressive behaviors.

Men tend to have less anxiety and thus they tend to get themselves into more trouble. In my lectures I often talk about the need for "enough" anxiety. For example, if someone gets the thought, "I think I'll go rob the grocery store," the very next thought should be "That's a very bad idea; you'll spend the next twenty years in jail." Some anxiety keeps you out of trouble. Too much, of course, can make you sick.

Hour 2 Exercise—Recruit Your Team and Make Your Worries Work for You

1. RECRUIT YOUR TEAM

Collaboration is a significant advantage of the female brain. To truly optimize your brain, you need a group of like-minded women to help.

THE STRENGTHS AND CHALLENGES
OF THE FEMALE BRAIN

Strengths

Longevity

Takes physical and mental health more seriously

Admits problems faster

Seeks help and community support faster

Worries more about her health

Exhibits lower incidence of too-little anxiety, a condition that can get her into trouble

Is more likely to sign up for health programs

Is more compliant in following brain-healthy recommendations, as demonstrated in the Amen Clinics outcome study

Is less likely to be in the "don't worry, be happy" group that dies early

Engages in fewer high-risk behaviors, thereby resulting in a healthier brain

Has stronger PFC, associated with greater judgment, empathy, and self-control

Exhibits lower incidence of ADD, autism, substance abuse, antisocial behavior, and going to prison

Challenges

Exhibits lower serotonin levels

Worries more

Has trouble turning off her brain

Is always thinking, thinking, thinking

Repeats the same issue again and again

Focuses too much on problems, even when they are not there

Struggles more with sleep and feels pain more acutely

Exhibits higher incidence of anxiety, depression, body image issues, eating disorders, physical stress symptoms, and perfectionism

In the first half of this hour, your task is to find and convince two other women to do this program with you. Have them get a copy of the book or get it for them. If you do these exercises with a small group of like-minded women, you will dramatically improve your own success at boosting the power of your female brain. In medical school we often had the saying of "See one, do one, teach one." It is in the teaching where you always learn the most.

2. MAKE YOUR WORRIES WORK FOR YOU

Studies show that journaling is a powerful tool to help get worries under control and out of your head. One of the most important exercises I give my patients is to have them journal to manage their worries. It is a really simple, powerful exercise.

Whenever you get a worry (a negative thought that won't go away), write it down. The act of writing helps to crystallize it and get it out of your head. The worry is now on the paper, a tablet, computer, or phone. Once the worry is written, evaluate it for its accuracy. Is it true or realistic? If not, smile and let it stay on the paper to get it out of your head. If the worry has merit, write down three or four things you can do about the worry, and equally important, write down what you cannot do about the worry.

For example, Jeanne had a daughter, Nina, with developmental delays and many medical problems. Writing down her worries, and working through them was very helpful for her.

I worry Nina will not develop normally, that she will get sick and
die, and that I will not be a good enough mother.
What can I do about these worries?
Get Nina the proper medical care.
Be on the lookout online for new resources to help her. Nurture her
the best way I can.

Enlist my support group (husband, family, and church members to help).

What I can't do about it?

I cannot fix her.

I cannot will her to be well.

I can't make myself sick, as I will be no good for Nina.

3

ADOPT THE AMEN CLINICS METHOD FOR OPTIMIZING THE FEMALE BRAIN

KNOW YOUR BRAIN, IMPORTANT NUMBERS, AND THE FOUR CIRCLES FOR ULTIMATE SUCCESS

Having a very clear, Four Circles plan to boost your brain is the third step to unleashing the power of the female brain. The truth will set you free. But first, it will piss you off.

—GLORIA STEINEM

Annette had called our clinics because her twenty-three-year-old daughter Katie had gotten a dismal score on the Law School Admission Test (LSAT). Katie had dreamed of being a lawyer like her older sister, but she did not do well on exams owing to the intense anxiety she felt every time she took a test. Katie felt anxious at other times as well. Whenever Katie faced a significant challenge, such as a test or a job interview, she predicted failure. Her worry often caused her to spin out of control when she studied, which kept her from absorbing information that she was intellectually able to master. She frequently felt tense and struggled with numerous physical stress symptoms, including headaches, back pain, and stomach problems.

All of these symptoms worried Annette, who learned about our clinics from a friend whose daughter had been nearly thrown off the basketball team for temper outbursts. Through our help, that young woman was able to control her temper and lead her team to the state championship.

Annette's mother hoped that we could help Katie too, although she had already taken her to three psychiatrists, a couple of psychologists, and the school counselor. None of these professionals had been able to make significant inroads into Katie's anxiety, and Katie was feeling hopeless about her future. Using a very clear method, we were able to boost Katie's brain and improve every aspect of her life. She ultimately did much better on the LSAT and entered law school. This is the same approach you can use to boost your brain, even if you never suffer from anxiety or other mental health challenge. It is the Amen Clinics approach to change your brain and your life.

To truly unleash the power of your female brain, you need to make sure your brain is in the best shape possible.

THE AMEN CLINICS METHOD

Our largest referral network for the Amen Clinics is from our own patients and their families. Over the last twenty-two years at the Amen Clinics, we have seen tens of thousands of patients from all fifty states and ninety countries. The reason people come from all over the world for help is that our process is very different from our colleagues' in mental health. We believe it is essential to thoroughly evaluate the brain before trying to change it. "How do you know unless you look?" is a mantra we've been repeating for over two decades.

In a large six-month outcome study that we performed on our patients at Amen Clinics, 83 percent reported high levels of improvement in their quality of life and similarly high levels of improvements in depression and anxiety scores. The numbers were even better for our patients who were highly compliant with what we asked them to do.

Our goal in running the clinics is to study what we do to continually improve our ability to help the people we serve. Certainly not everyone who comes to one of our clinics gets better. There is still so much to learn, but compared to the published outcome studies in mental health, our success rates are exciting.

The knowledge we have obtained to help our patients can also help you be your best, whether you or a loved one suffer with a mental health issue, traumatic brain injury, PTSD, or you simply want to optimize the health of your brain. Unleashing the full power of your female brain starts by following our very clear method for success:

- Develop an in-depth understanding of where you are, using the Four Circles Approach, which assesses your biological, psychological, social, and spiritual health.

The method looks like this:

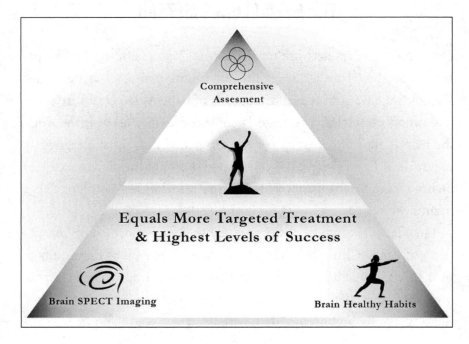

- Gather current information on how your brain functions, through brain SPECT imaging or computerized tests and questionnaires.
- Know your important health numbers, including standard lab tests to make sure your body is functioning properly (your brain and body are interconnected).
- Target help specifically to your vulnerable areas.
- Engage in regular brain-healthy habits.

So let's break down this method and, as an instructive example, apply it to Katie's life. Apply it to yours as well.

THE AMEN CLINICS FOUR CIRCLES APPROACH: A BIO/PSYCHO/SOCIAL/SPIRITUAL ASSESSMENT

When I was a first-year medical student at Oral Roberts University in Tulsa, Oklahoma, our dean, Dr. Sid Garrett, gave us one of our first lectures on how to help people of any age for any problem. That lecture has stayed with me for the last thirty-five years. Dr. Garrett told us, "Always think of people as whole beings, never just as their symptoms." He insisted that whenever we evaluated anyone, we should take into consideration the four circles:

- **Biology:** how the physical body functions
- **Psychology:** developmental issues and thought patterns
- **Social connections:** social support and current life situation
- **Spiritual health:** what life means

At the Amen Clinics we use these four circles to take a balanced, comprehensive approach to healing. These principles have impacted my own life and career, and once you really understand them, they can help you get and stay powerful in the most balanced way possible.

THE AMEN CLINICS FOUR CIRCLES OF POWER, HEALTH, AND HEALING

UNDERSTANDING YOUR VULNERABILITIES

BIOLOGY/BODY PSYCHOLOGY/MIND

- Brain health
- Overall physical health
- Nutrition
- Exercise
- Sleep
- Hydration
- Hormones
- Blood sugar level
- Nutritional supplementation
- Genetics – family history
- Trauma/injuries
- Allergies (food, mold, etc.)
- Toxins (environment (mold), drugs, alcohol, excessive caffeine, smoking)
- Infections
- Physical illness
- Medication

- How we talk to ourselves
- Self-concept
- Body image
- Upbringing
- Developmental issues
- Past emotional trauma
- Past successes
- Past failures
- Grief
- Generational histories and issues (i.e., immigrants, survivors of trauma, children/ grandchildren of alcoholics)
- Hope
- Sense of worth
- Sense of power or control

BIOLOGY

Your biology comprises the first circle of health, illness, and optimization: the physical aspects of your brain and body and how they function together. For your biology to operate at peak efficiency, its machinery (cells, connections, chemicals, energy, blood flow, and waste processing) needs to work right. The brain is like a supercomputer, with both hardware and software. Think of your biology as your hardware. Within the biology circle are factors such as your genetics, overall physical health, nutrition, exercise, sleep, and hormones, as well as environmental issues, such as toxins. When the brain's biology is healthy, all of these factors work together in a positive way to maximize your success. When trauma, toxins, illness, or deficiencies affect your biology, you feel disrupted or out of sync.

For example, when you don't get enough sleep, you have overall decreased blood flow to your brain, which disrupts thinking, memory, and concentration. Likewise, a brain injury hurts the machinery of the brain, causing you to struggle with depression, memory issues, and temper problems. When you eat a high-sugar or simple-carbohydrate diet, your blood sugar often becomes dysregulated, causing you to feel sluggish and foggy-headed.

KATIE'S BIOLOGY

Katie's biology played a significant role in her anxiety and her resulting poor performance on tests. She had a family history of panic disorder, which is a highly heritable problem and is associated with a tendency toward anxiety. Katie's mother and grandfather struggled with anxiety, and she had an aunt who suffered from panic disorder with agoraphobia and didn't leave her house for fifteen years.

Katie's anxiety was made worse by other biological factors. Katie rarely slept more than six hours at night, which has been shown in many studies to affect learning and mood. In addition, Katie's diet, like that of many twenty-three-year-olds, consisted of a lot of junk food and caffeinated drinks as she tried to stay alert. She rarely exercised, drank more alcohol than she admitted to her mother, and struggled with intestinal problems.

At age five, Katie's mother had gotten into an accident in which she rolled the car five times. Katie had been in the car and had almost certainly received a brain injury that affected her development. Significantly, her high-performing sister had not been in the accident.

I explained to Katie and her mother that an essential part of being her best was to bring these biological factors into balance: healing past injuries and protecting herself from future injuries; getting good sleep; avoiding toxins, such as drugs or excessive alcohol; eating a healthy, balanced diet; getting plenty of exercise; and taking fish oil, a multiple vitamin, and any targeted supplements or medications that may be needed. Without biological interventions, I told them, Katie would never perform at her best. Of course, with *only* biological interventions, especially if all I did for Katie was to medicate her anxiety, her improvement would not be nearly as robust as if she followed through in all four circles.

PSYCHOLOGY

Psychological factors fall into the second circle of health, illness, and optimization. This circle includes how we think and talk to ourselves, the running dialogue that goes on in our minds, as well as our self-concept, body image, past traumas, overall upbringing, and significant developmental events. Being raised in a reasonably happy home, getting positive messages growing up, and feeling comfortable with our abilities and our bodies all contribute to psychological health. When we struggle in any of these areas, we are less likely to be successful. If we perceive ourselves as unattractive or less able than our peers, trouble starts to brew. If our thinking patterns are excessively negative, harsh, or critical, that will have a negative impact on our moods, anxiety levels, and ultimately on our ability to function successfully.

Developmental issues, such as being adopted or experiencing a significant loss or trauma as a child, are also significant. Children often believe that they are the center of the universe and that if something bad happens, such as if a mother gets cancer, a child may think it is her fault and spend the rest of her life wracked with guilt. Past successes and failures are a part of this circle, as are hope and a sense of worth and personal power or control.

Generational histories can also be very important in the psyche of a developing brain. Children of immigrants or Holocaust survivors often get very different psychological messages from those of children whose families have been established for generations. For example, many Holocaust survivors will never speak to their children or grandchildren about what happened. Nonetheless, the messages of the unspeakable horrors may be transmitted nonverbally to the subsequent generations, and the younger generations can end up with anxiety and PTSD issues without ever hearing the actual stories. The trauma messages can be conveyed unconsciously through looks and gestures.

KATIE'S PSYCHOLOGY

Katie had an undisciplined mind. Her negative thoughts about impending failure controlled her mood and frightened her on a regular basis. It was as if she had a roving band of thugs in her head, taunting her by predicting the worst outcomes for her life.

Katie had an infestation of ANTs going on between her ears. In addition, she had a negative self-concept about learning, because school had been hard for her. Because she was unaware of the anxiety issue and potential head trauma issue, Katie thought that she was a lazy person who was just not very smart, even though she tried harder than any of her siblings. Because her parents didn't understand the situation, they assumed Katie wasn't making much of an effort. They often told her to try harder, which, of course, didn't help.

In fact, the more pressure Katie felt, the worse she performed. The competition with her older sister was painful and she always believed she could never live up to her sibling's success.

As for all of us, understanding her psychological issues and learning not to believe every stupid thought she had was an essential part of Katie's road to recovery, and a key aspect of the treatment plan I gave her.

SOCIAL CONNECTIONS

The social connections circle of health, illness, and optimization emphasizes the current relationships and events in our lives. When we are in good relationships, experience good health, have a job we love, school we care about, and enough money, our brain tends to do much better than when any of these areas stress or trouble us. Stress negatively impacts brain function, and dealing with difficult events makes us more vulnerable to illness. Depression is often triggered by current stressful life events, such as marital problems, family dysfunction, financial difficulties, health problems, work- or school-related struggles, or losses. Plus, the health and habits of the people you spend time with have a dramatic impact on your own health and habits.

KATIE'S SOCIAL CONNECTIONS

Katie felt constant stress about the LSAT and getting into law school. In addition, she was fighting with her boyfriend, who she felt didn't understand her. Her parents tried to soothe her, but it never seemed to take. In fact, the more they tried to soothe her, the more anxious and frantic Katie became.

Sometimes it seemed to Katie that *everything* stressed her: her family, her boyfriend, the LSAT, and the prospect of law school. Katie was working as an administrative assistant to save money for school, but she felt stressed by that job too, which often required mandatory overtime and cut into Katie's social life and study time in unpredictable ways. Katie worried about getting fired and not being able to get another job. "How can I, if my boss won't recommend me?" she asked me. Katie had a hard time distinguishing between her worst fears (*I will get fired and my boss might not give me a recommendation*) and reality (*Sometimes my boss is annoyed with me, but mainly she appreciates what I do for her and will not fire me or give me a bad reference*).

Typical for an anxious person, Katie's constant worries seemed impossible to resolve. After talking to Katie for hours, her parents, boyfriend, or girlfriends might make small progress, but usually within an hour or two after the conversation, Katie would go right back to feeling anxious.

Optimizing Katie's present life, including helping her manage stress and effectively deal with her relationships, was an essential part of her treatment plan. Since decreasing the daily stress in your life also improves brain function, I told Katie that regular stress-management techniques were crucial for her overall brain health and for unleashing the power of her female brain.

SPIRITUAL HEALTH

Beyond the biological, psychological, and social aspects our lives, we are also spiritual beings. So to fully heal and recover, we must recognize that we are more than just our bodies, minds, and social connections, and we must ask ourselves deep spiritual questions, such as the following:

> What does my life mean?
> What is my purpose?
> Why am I here?
> What are my values?
> Do I believe in God or a Higher Power?
> How does that manifest in my life?
> What is my connection to past generations, future
>   generations, and the planet?

Having a sense of purpose, as well as connections to past and future generations, allows us to reach beyond ourselves to affirm that our lives matter. Without a spiritual connection, many people experience an overriding sense of despair. Morality, values, and a spiritual connection to others and the universe are critical for many people to feel a sense of wholeness and connection, and a reason to get up in the morning and to take good care of themselves.

KATIE'S SPIRITUAL HEALTH

Katie had never really asked herself why she was here or why her life mattered. She hadn't even thought about what her life might be like five, ten, or fifty years down the road. As for many young adults, the present moment was what mattered to Katie, not the future. Getting her to think beyond the moment and get in touch with her sense of purpose and meaning was crucial to her unleashing the power of her female brain, and it is crucial for you too.

GET YOUR BRAIN ASSESSED

You can do a great job assessing your four circles but still not fully optimize your brain. You also need to understand how your brain functions. At the Amen Clinics, we have three ways to evaluate brain function:

1. Brain SPECT imaging
2. Questionnaires
3. Online assessments

BRAIN SPECT IMAGING

As mentioned earlier, we do a study called brain SPECT imaging, which looks at blood flow and activity patterns. SPECT gives a direct look at how the brain works. SPECT scans are actually easy to understand because we basically look for three things:

· Areas of the brain that work well (normal activity)
· Areas of the brain that work too hard (high activity)
· Areas of the brain that do not work hard enough (low activity)

A healthy SPECT scan shows full, even, symmetrical activity, with the highest activity in the cerebellum, which is located in the back, bottom part of the brain. In demonstrating SPECT scans at lectures, I generally show them in two views: an outside *surface* scan view, that helps us see low areas of activity, and an *active* scan view, which shows us areas of the brain that are working too hard. As I mentioned, women tend to have much busier brains than men.

SPECT scans help us see vulnerable areas that need to be optimized, even years before trouble may actually show itself. It is now thought that functional imaging studies like SPECT show evidence of Alzheimer's disease, a form of dementia, years before people have any symptoms. It is not just by helping us recognize dementia and memory problems that SPECT can help. In a scientific study we published last year, getting a SPECT scan changed either the diagnosis or treatment plan in nearly eight out of ten patients. Having a scan helps us see more clearly what is happening in the brain that may be the cause of someone's emotional and cognitive struggles, such as undiagnosed brain injuries (22 percent) or toxic exposure (22 percent).

SPECT scans also help us see someone's strengths and vulnerabilities. For example, if they have a tendency toward impulse control problems, we are more likely to see low activity in the PFC, located in the front part of the brain. If they tend to be rigid and inflexible, we often see increased activity in an area of the frontal part of the brain called the anterior cingulate gyrus.

Researchers from Japan found that brain blood flow in certain areas of the brain was positively correlated with both intelligence and creativity. Protecting the brain's blood flow is critical to having a healthy mind.

Besides helping us make more complete diagnoses, SPECT helps lead us to direct treatment in the context of a bio/psycho/social/spiritual assessment. Without a scan or another measure of brain function, it is like throwing darts in the dark at someone's brain. If you visit the Amen Clinics website (www.amenclinics.com), you can see hundreds of brain SPECT scans and read over twenty-six hundred scientific abstracts on SPECT for a wide variety of behavioral, mood, learning, and mental health issues.

Nine Ways SPECT Will Change Everything You Do

1. You Will Develop Brain Envy—Upon seeing her scan, forty-five-year-old Betsy knew she had to get healthy. She had problems with drinking and drug abuse after being in an emotionally traumatic relationship. After seeing her scan, however, she developed brain envy and completely changed her habits. A year later her brain looked much better.

Betsy

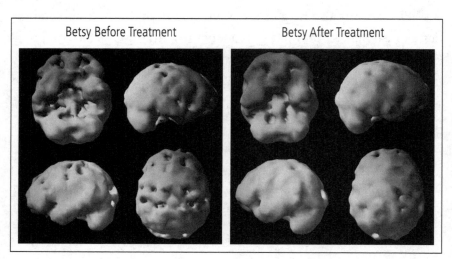

| Betsy Before Treatment | Betsy After Treatment |

2. You Will Be Careful with Many Psychotropic Medications—I am a classically trained psychiatrist and have used medications to help my patients for many years. However, when I started ordering scans, I saw that some medication classes like benzodiazepines (antianxiety medications) and opiate painkillers made the brain look toxic, like our alcoholics' brains. It was then I started looking for natural ways to heal the brain.

Healthy Scan vs. Benzodiazepine Scan

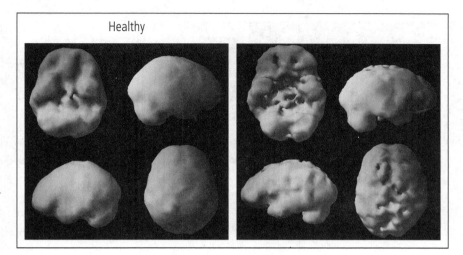

Healthy

Chronic Benzodiazepine Use

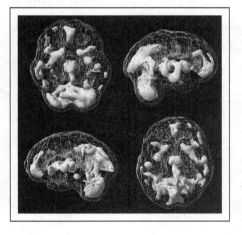

3. You Won't Let Your Kids Play Tackle Football or Hit Soccer Balls with Their Heads—The brain is soft and the skull is hard with many sharp bony ridges. Brain injuries matter and ruin people's brains and their lives.

NFL Player

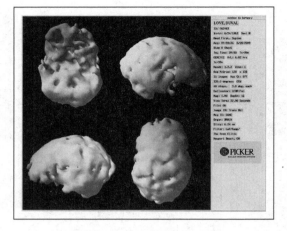

4. You Will Take Sleep Apnea More Seriously—On a SPECT scan, sleep apnea, a condition in which a person snores loudly, stops breathing at night, and is often chronically tired during the day, makes the brain appear very low in activity. Sleep apnea doubles a person's risk for getting Alzheimer's. If you have any symptoms, make sure to have your physician order a sleep study.

Sleep apnea

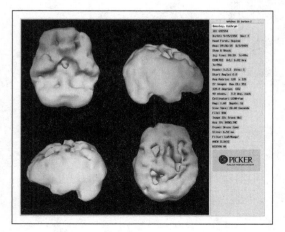

5. You Will Take Your Weight More Seriously—There are eighteen studies now that report that as your weight goes up, the actual physical size and function of your brain go down. That should just scare the fat off all of us. Below is one of my patients with morbid obesity.

Obesity Scan

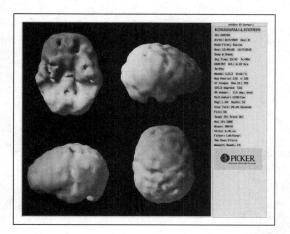

6. You Will See That There Is Not a One-Size-Fits-All Treatment for Depression and Other Illnesses—Based on our im-

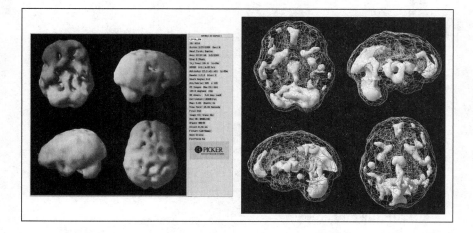

aging work, we have discovered that illnesses like ADD, anxiety, depression, and addictions are not single or simple illness in the brain; they all have multiple types and thus multiple treatments.

7. You Will Start Thinking About the Early Detection and Prevention of Alzheimer's Disease—SPECT scans show trouble years before people have any symptoms of memory problems. Scans alert you when a problem may be brewing in the brain.

Early Alzheimer's

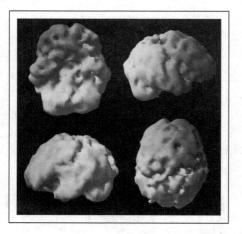

8. You Will Work Harder Not to Call People Bad Names— When people act badly, it is easy to just call them negative or derogatory names. But once you look at their scans and realize they might have a damaged or toxic scan, it gives you more understanding and empathy.

Toxic Brain Damage

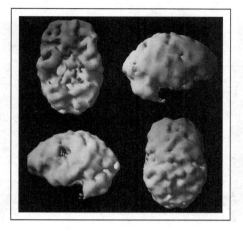

9. You Will Think About the Brain if You Are Having Relationship Problems—I have looked at the scans of over a thousand couples who are having serious relationship problems. Often, one or both of the partners has a brain challenge that no one is aware of. Helping to heal and optimize the brain helps people get along better with others.

Brain Injury

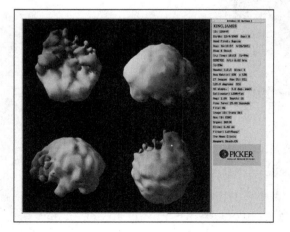

KATIE'S SPECT SCANS

Katie's SPECT Scans Low Activity

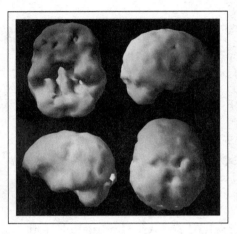

Katie's SPECT Scans High Activity

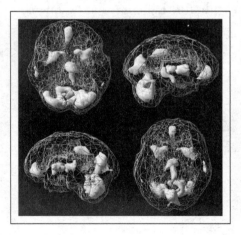

Katie's scans showed several important findings, including a mild brain injury pattern to the left side of her brain, which likely resulted from the car accident. She also showed high activity in the anxiety and worry centers of her brain, which was consistent with the anxiety issues she had reported. These findings made the need to heal the past brain injury and treat her anxiety even clearer.

AMEN SOLUTION BRAIN TYPE QUESTIONNAIRE

Unfortunately, not everyone is able to get a scan, either because of cost or a lack of availability in your area. My books are translated into thirty languages, so if you read one in China or Brazil, odds are you're not going to come to one of our Amen Clinics to get a scan and evaluation. So, based on thousands of scans, I developed a series of questionnaires to help people predict what their scans might look like if they *could* get one. The questionnaires are not as individually precise as the scans, especially when there are complex issues involved, but many people find them very helpful, and they are used by thousands of mental health professionals around the world.

You can take our Amen Solution Brain Type Questionnaire on our web coaching site, the Amen Solution @ Home (www.amensolution .com). The questionnaire will help you evaluate your brain's function in the following areas:

- Flexible thinking
- Focus/impulse control
- Mood
- Stress and anxiety
- Memory
- Sleep
- Cravings
- Brain-healthy habits

Based on your answers, we give targeted recommendations, including science-based natural ways to boost the brain. Of course, it is important to talk to your health care provider about any recommendations.

24/7 BRAIN GYM ASSESSMENT

Also, on the Amen Solution @ Home site, we have a 24/7 Brain Gym, where you can test and work out your brain at any time. It starts with a sophisticated thirty-minute computerized assessment to determine the health of your brain. It measures mood, attention span, impulse control, memory, reaction time, and more. Based on your score, the program will give you exercises tailored to enhance your specific brain. Spending ten minutes a day in the 24/7 Brain Gym is a great way to unleash the power of your female brain by boosting your brain power!

KATIE'S QUESTIONNAIRE AND 24/7 BRAIN GYM RESULTS

Katie's questionnaire showed likely problems with stress, anxiety, and inflexible thinking. The results from her brain assessment also showed evidence of anxiety and stress and were consistent with her scan. The online program gave her very specific exercises to calm her anxiety and begin to help her correct the negative thinking patterns. For example, it recommended one of my favorite games, "E-Catch the Feeling." In this brain exercise, bubbles are shot in the air with "positive" words, such *as joy, happiness, success,* and *relaxation,* and "negative" words, such as *despair, anger, frustration,* and *sadness.* The task is to click on the positive words and ignore the negative ones. This game has been found to help focus people's thoughts in a more positive direction. The assessment also recommended another game, "MyCalmBeat," which taught Katie to breathe in a way to optimize the feeling of relaxation and well-being.

I knew that the Four Circles Approach, brain assessments, and other tools could help Katie get back on track.

KNOW YOUR IMPORTANT NUMBERS

Another very important part of optimizing your brain is to know your important health numbers. I often say you cannot change what you do not measure. Here is the list of the key numbers you should know about yourself:

1. Body mass index (BMI)
2. Waist-to-height ratio (WHtR)
3. Average hours slept each night and an assessment of whether you have sleep apnea
4. Blood pressure

1. Body Mass Index—The BMI is a measure of your weight compared to your height. A normal BMI is between 18.5 and 24.9. Overweight is between 25 and 30. Obese is greater than 30. You can find a simple BMI calculator on the web.

Knowing your BMI is important because being overweight or obese has been associated with less brain tissue and lower brain activity. Obesity doubles the risk for Alzheimer's disease and depression. There are probably several mechanisms that create this result, including the fact that fat cells produce inflammatory chemicals and store toxic materials in the body. I want you to know your BMI, because it stops you from lying to yourself about your weight.

2. Waist-to-Height Ratio—Another way to measure the health of your weight is by using the WHtR. Some researchers believe this number is even more accurate than BMI. The WHtR is calculated by dividing waist size by height. For an example, a female with a 32-inch waist who is 5 feet 10 inches (70 inches) would divide 32 by 70 to get a WHtR of 45.7 percent. To be healthy your waist size in inches should be less than half your height. So, if you are 66 inches tall, your waist should not be more than 33 inches. If you are 72 inches tall, your waist should not be more than 36 inches.

The WHtR is thought to give a more accurate assessment of health since the most dangerous place to carry weight is in the abdomen. Fat in the abdomen, which is associated with a larger waist, is metabolically active and produces various hormones that can cause harmful effects, such as diabetes, elevated blood pressure, and high cholesterol and triglyceride levels.

Note: *You have to actually measure your waist size with a tape measure!* Going by your pants size does not count, as many clothing manufacturers actually make their sizes larger than they state on the label so as not to offend their customers. In my experience, 90 percent of people will underestimate their waist circumference. Don't lie to yourself.

3. The Number of Hours You Sleep Each Night—One of the fastest ways to hurt your brain is to get fewer than seven or eight hours of sleep at night. People who typically get six hours or fewer of sleep have lower overall blood flow to the brain, which hurts its function. Researchers from the Walter Reed Army Institute of Research and the University of Pennsylvania found that chronically getting fewer than eight hours of sleep was associated with cognitive decline. Strive to get at least seven or eight hours of sleep a night. There are hypnosis audios on the Amen Solution @ Home.

Chronic insomnia triples your risk of death from all causes.

4. Blood Pressure—To keep your brain healthy, it is critical to know your blood pressure. High blood pressure is associated with lower overall brain function, which means more bad decisions. Here are the numbers you should know:

Optimal blood pressure: below 120/80
Prehypertension:120/80–139/89
Hypertension: 140 (or above) / 90 (or above)

Check your blood pressure or have your doctor check it on a regular basis. If your blood pressure is high, make sure to take it seriously. Some behaviors that can help lower your blood pressure include losing weight, daily exercise, fish oil supplements, and if needed, medication.

GET YOUR WEIGHT UNDER CONTROL: FEED YOUR BRAIN RIGHT

You'll find a detailed explanation of the optimal way to feed your female brain to attain and maintain your optimal weight in chapter 5. You can also find more suggestions for a brain-healthy diet on our website (www.amensolution.com), as well as loads of delicious brain-healthy recipes.

KATIE'S IMPORTANT NUMBERS

Katie's weight was normal and her blood pressure was fine, but her sleep habits were not good. Her anxiety kept her from sleeping, and the lack of sleep made her more anxious. It was a vicious cycle that needed to be stopped.

GET KEY LABORATORY TESTS

Laboratory tests are the next set of important numbers to know. Here are the key lab test numbers you need to know:

1. Complete blood count
2. General metabolic panel with fasting blood sugar and lipid panel
3. HgA1C
4. Vitamin D
5. Thyroid panel
6. C-reactive protein
7. Homocysteine
8. Ferritin

9. Free and total serum testosterone

10. Cortisol and sulfated DHEA (DHEA-S)

11. Estrogen and progesterone

These tests can be ordered by your health care professional, or you can order them for yourself on websites such as SaveOnLabs.com.

1. Complete Blood Count (blood test)—This test checks the health of your blood, including red and white blood cells. People with low blood count can feel anxious and tired, and they can have significant memory problems.

2. General Metabolic Panel with Fasting Blood Sugar and Lipid Panel (blood test)—This test checks the health of your liver, kidneys, fasting blood sugar, cholesterol, and triglycerides. Fasting blood sugar is especially important. Normal is between 70 and 90 mg/dL (milligrams per deciliter); prediabetes is between 91 and 125 mg/dL; and diabetes is 126 mg/dL or higher. According to a large study from Kaiser Permanente, for every point above 85, patients had an additional 6 percent increased risk of developing diabetes in the next ten years (87 = 12 percent increased risk, 88 = 18 percent increased risk, etc.). Above 90 indicates that vascular damage has already occurred and a patient is at risk for having damage to the kidneys and eyes.

Why is high fasting blood sugar a problem? High blood sugar causes vascular problems throughout your whole body, including your brain. Over time, it causes blood vessels to become brittle and vulnerable to breakage. It leads not only to diabetes but also to heart disease, strokes, visual impairment, impaired wound healing, wrinkled skin, and cognitive problems. Diabetes doubles the risk for Alzheimer's disease.

Cholesterol and triglycerides are also important. Sixty percent of the solid weight of the brain is fat. High cholesterol is obviously bad for the brain, but having it too low is also bad, as some cholesterol is essential to make sex hormones and help the brain function properly. According to the American Heart Association, optimal levels are as follows:

- Total cholesterol (135–200 mg/dL, below 135 has been associated with depression)
- High-density lipoprotein (HDL) (>= 60 mg/dL)
- Low-density lipoprotein (LDL) (@100 mg/dL)
- Triglycerides (@100 mg/Dl)

If your lipids are off, make sure to get your diet under control, as well as taking fish oil and exercising regularly. Of course you should see your physician. Also, knowing the particle size of LDL cholesterol is important. Large particles are less toxic than smaller particles.

3. HgA1C (blood test)—This test shows your average blood sugar levels over the past two to three months and is used to diagnose diabetes and prediabetes. Normal results for a nondiabetic person are in the 4–5.6 percent range. Prediabetes is indicated by levels in the 5.7–6.4 percent range. Higher numbers may indicate diabetes.

4. Vitamin D (blood test)—Low levels of vitamin D have been associated with obesity, depression, cognitive impairment, heart disease, reduced immunity, cancer, psychosis, and all causes of mortality. Check your 25-hydroxy vitamin D level, and if it is low, try get more sunshine in a safe way and/or take a vitamin D_3 supplement. A healthy vitamin D level is between 30 and 100 ng/dL (nanograms per deciliter). Optimal is between 50 and 100 ng/

dL. Personally, I never wanted to be in the bottom of any class I was ever in. Two-thirds of the population are low in vitamin D; this is the same percentage of U.S. residents who are overweight or obese. According to one study, when vitamin D is low the hormone leptin that tells us to stop eating is not effective. One of the reasons for the dramatic rise in vitamin D deficiency is that people are wearing more sunscreen and spending more time inside working or in front of the television or computer.

5. Thyroid Panel (blood test)—Abnormal thyroid hormone levels are a common cause of anxiety, depression, forgetfulness, confusion, and lethargy. Having low thyroid levels decreases overall brain activity, which can impair your thinking, judgment, and self-control and make it very hard for you to feel good. Low thyroid functioning can make it nearly impossible to manage weight effectively. To know your thyroid levels, you need to know these figures:

- thyroid-stimulating hormone (TSH)
- Free T3
- Free T4
- Thyroid antibodies (thyroid peroxidase and thyroglobulin antibodies)

There is no one perfect way, no one symptom or test result, that will properly diagnose low thyroid function or hypothyroidism. The key is to look at your symptoms and your blood tests, and then decide. Symptoms of low thyroid include fatigue; depression; mental fog; dry skin; hair loss, especially the outer third of your eyebrows; feeling cold when others feel normal, constipation; hoarse voice; and weight gain. Most doctors do not check thyroid antibodies unless the TSH is high. This is a big mistake. Many people have autoimmunity against their thyroid, which makes it function poorly, even while they still have a "normal" TSH. That's why I think measuring the antibodies should also be part of routine screening.

6.C-Reactive Protein (blood test)—This is a measure of inflammation. Elevated inflammation is associated with a number of diseases and conditions that are associated with mood problems, aging, and cognitive impairment. Fat cells produce chemicals that increase inflammation. A healthy range is between 0.0 and 1.0 mg/dL. This is a very good test for inflammation. It measures the general level of inflammation although it does not tell you what has caused this condition.

The most common reason for an elevated C-reactive protein is metabolic syndrome or insulin resistance. The second most common is some sort of reaction to food, either a true allergy, a food sensitivity, or an autoimmune reaction such as occurs with gluten. High levels of C-reactive protein can also indicate hidden infections. You'll learn more about how to detect and overcome food reactions in chapter 5.

7. Homocysteine (blood test)—Elevated homocysteine levels (>10 mmol/L, or micromoles per liter) in the blood have been associated with damage to the lining of arteries and atherosclerosis (hardening and narrowing of the arteries) as well as an increased risk of heart attacks, strokes, blood clot formation, and possibly Alzheimer's disease. This is a sensitive marker for B vitamin deficiency, including folic acid deficiency. Replacing these vitamins often helps return the homocysteine level to normal.

8. Ferritin (blood test)—This is a measure of iron stores, a number that increases with inflammation and insulin resistance. Levels between 15 and 200 ng/mL for females are ideal. Women tend to have lower iron stores than men, owing to blood loss from years of menstruation, since blood cells contain iron. Some theorize that this is one of the reasons that women live longer than men.

However, you don't want ferritin levels that are too low, as this is associated with anemia, restless legs, ADD, and low motivation and energy. Higher iron stores have been associated with stiffer blood vessels and vascular disease. Some research suggests that donating blood to lower high ferritin levels may enhance blood vessel flexibility and help decrease the risk of heart disease. Plus, whenever you give blood you are being altruistic, which is also good for your mind and body.

9. Free and Total Serum Testosterone (blood test)—For both men and women, low levels of testosterone have been associated with low energy, cardiovascular disease, obesity, low libido, depression, and Alzheimer's disease. Normal levels for adult females are:

· Total testosterone in females (30–95 ng/dL)
· Free testosterone in females (0.4–1.9 ng/dL)

10. Cortisol (saliva test) and DHEA-S (blood test)—These adrenal gland hormones are related to stress, and DHEA is a precursor to other hormones. In the blood I measure cortisol (11–14 μg /dL is optimal) and DHEA-S. Most normal lab values are between 5 and 25, but you're not striving for normal here; you want optimal numbers. If I want to know more about cortisol, I will measure cortisol four times a day (morning, noon, dinner, and bedtime) using saliva.

11. Estrogen and Progesterone—These are measured depending on the circumstances in blood or saliva. When menstruating, they are usually measured on day 21 of the cycle; after menopause, they can be measured any time. Estrogen is responsible for vaginal lubrication, helps with libido, aids in memory, and so much more. Progesterone calms emotions, creates a restful sleep, and acts as a diuretic. There is much more on hormones in the next chapter.

BOOSTING YOUR BRAIN

If your results on any of these tests are less than optimal, follow the suggestions in this book, and also see your health care provider about specific solutions.

KNOW YOUR TWELVE MODIFIABLE HEALTH-RISK FACTORS

Know how many of the twelve most important modifiable health risk factors you have, then work to decrease them. Here is a list of these factors compiled by researchers at the Harvard School of Public Health. Circle the ones that apply to you.

1. Smoking
2. High blood pressure
3. Being overweight or obese
4. Physical inactivity
5. High fasting blood glucose
6. High LDL cholesterol
7. Alcohol abuse (accidents, injuries, violence, cirrhosis, liver disease, cancer, stroke, heart disease, hypertension)
8. Low omega-3 fatty acids
9. High dietary saturated fat intake
10. Low polyunsaturated fat intake
11. High dietary salt
12. Low intake of fruits and vegetables

KATIE'S LABORATORY TESTS

Katie's numbers showed that her diet and lifestyle choices were almost certainly contributing to her brain problems. Although her weight was in the healthy range, she often struggled with getting eight hours of sleep. She had a low vitamin D level, and she had a low intake of fruits and vegetables. Because of her high consumption of fast foods, she had a high intake of dietary salt and saturated fats, along with few omega-3 fatty acids in her diet. Plus, she was sedentary.

I knew that cleaning up Katie's diet and improving her sleep would ease her anxiety and improve her mood. Altering these elements of her biology would go a long way toward boosting Katie's brain and unleashing its power.

TARGETED HELP FOR YOUR VULNERABLE AREAS

Once you have completed the Four Circles Approach, analyzed the health of your brain systems, noted your important numbers, and gotten the key laboratory tests, you are ready to get healthier than ever in your life by developing a personalized, targeted plan that addresses your biology, psychology, social connections, and spiritual health. When you look at people through the lens of brain imaging, you realize that a one-size-fits-all approach to treatment makes no sense. The program needs to be tailored or personalized to your specific brain and body.

TARGETED HELP FOR KATIE

The Amen Clinics Method of integrated care was extremely helpful to Katie. Based on what we found from Katie's assessments, brain scans, questionnaires, key numbers, and lab results, we created her individualized Four Circles treatment plan.

Biology—Here we focused on improving Katie's sleep, diet, and exercise habits. Katie agreed to cut out the alcohol and the caffeinated sodas and to get rid of the junk, focusing instead on brain-healthy food, filtered water, and decaffeinated green tea, all of which are terrific for boosting your brain.

We also discovered that Katie had two common food sensitivities to dairy and to gluten (found in wheat and other grains), so she cut out dairy products, wheat, barley, pasta, bread, and other items made with white flour. As you'll see in chapter 5, the intestinal tract is virtually a second brain. The gut makes more neurotransmitters than the brain. Neurotransmitters are key biochemicals that regulate mood and energy.

Within two weeks, Katie was more relaxed than she had been in years, and her intestinal problems were well on their way to clearing up. She also felt more focused and alert.

We also wanted to rehabilitate Katie's head injury. The first step here was helping Katie to develop brain envy. As soon as she was able to compare her scan to that of a healthy brain's, she reacted as so many people do, wanting to do whatever she could to care for her brain. She was ready to follow the brain-healthy habits I describe in the next section: Avoid anything that hurts your brain (bad food, insufficient sleep, chronic stress), and consistently do things that help your brain (eating well, sleeping well, and correcting any underlying negative thought patterns).

I also prescribed some simple dietary supplements for Katie. I believe that everyone needs a multivitamin (as most people do not eat at least five servings of vegetables and fruits a day) and about 2,000 mg fish oil, taken in supplement form. Katie's tests showed that she was low on vitamin D—most people are—so I suggested she take vitamin D supplements. I also suggested that Katie take probiotics, which support your digestion by replenishing healthy gut bacteria. And I gave Katie a special supplement I have designed that supports healthy serotonin levels to help her be less worried; I prescribed another one to help support overall brain function.

Psychology—Katie scored very high on the questionnaire that measured stress and anxiety and on the one that rated inflexible thinking. So it was very important to teach her the Amen Clinics ANT therapy to help her drive out the negative thoughts that kept automatically cropping up in her head. I'll teach you how to drive out the ANTs in chapter 6, or you can go to www.amensolution.com for more information.

I also wanted to make sure to expose Katie to the meditation and hypnosis audios on the Amen Solution @ Home website. Self-hypnosis and meditation are very helpful for anxiety, and Katie found that using these brain-healthy tools made her calmer and more focused right away. Katie also learned that when she felt stressed, she could soothe her brain by taking ten slow, deep breaths.

Finally, I talked to Katie about making good decisions. People often ask me, "What's the *one* thing I should do to boost my brain?" Start making better decisions today. How do you do that? Just plant in your mind these two little words: *Then what?*

"I think I'm going to stay up late tonight and answer emails." *Then what?* "Oh, if I do that, I'll be tired and crabby the next day, and I won't be able to enjoy that special family dinner we have planned. Instead, I'll go to bed and get some good sleep."

"I think I'll take a piece of that chocolate cake from the buffet." *Then what?* "Well, twenty minutes from now, I'll feel guilty, ashamed, and stupid. I don't like feeling that way! I guess I'll grab an apple and walk out so I won't be tempted." Keep these two words with you everywhere you go: *Then what?*

Social Connections—Like many stressed and anxious people, Katie tended to withdraw and isolate herself in times of trouble. I encouraged her to reach out when she was upset, to find someone she trusted, take a walk, and talk it out. Her parents, her boyfriend, and her girlfriends all became trusted members of Katie's support system.

Spiritual Health—In the Spiritual Health circle on p. 000, I list several questions for people to ask themselves. I encouraged Katie to really think about these questions, asking herself what her life meant, why she cared, and why the things that mattered to her were important. On our website, you will find a "One-Page Miracle" where you have the chance to think about what you truly want in your life in relationships, work, money, and for yourself. Katie completed this page, and that really got her thinking. She began spending time focusing on what her life means and what she wants her life to mean. She started each day reviewing her "One-Page Miracle" so that she could focus on the things that were really important to her.

The essence of mental health is knowing what you want and then being able to act in a way consistent with getting it. For example, I ask myself, "If I want a kind, caring relationship with my wife, what do I need to do to make that happen?" Katie asked herself, "If I want to get into law school, what do I need to do to make that happen?"

This question led Katie to realize that passing the LSAT was key to getting into law school, and not getting sick was key to passing her tests. Now she felt more motivation to boost her brain.

REGULAR BRAIN-HEALTHY HABITS

Developing regular brain-healthy habits is a critical piece in boosting your brain and unleashing its power. You must take your habits seriously and put habits into your life that serve you rather than steal from you. Through the years I have come up with an incredibly simple way to boost brain health. It really takes just three strategies:

1. *Develop brain envy.* You have to truly want to have a better brain.
2. *Avoid anything that hurts your brain.* **This includes** drugs, alcohol, environmental toxins, obesity, hypertension, diabetes, heart disease, sleep apnea, depression, negative thinking patterns, excessive stress, and a lack of exercise or new learning.
3. *Consistently do good behaviors that help your brain.* **Adopt** a great diet, learn new things, exercise, develop accurate thinking habits, work on stress management, and take some simple supplements to nourish your brain.

HIGH LEVELS OF SUCCESS

To be at your best, it is critical to put all of these pieces into place. Taking an integrated approach to boosting your brain gives you the best chance to feel great, look great, and to achieve your ideal weight.

Hour 3 Exercise—Get Assessed

Review the Four Circles—Make a copy of the Four Circles diagram on p. 000, and mark the areas in each circle that apply to you, to see your strengths and vulnerabilities

Take the Amen Solution Brain Type Test—Log on to the Amen Solution @ Home (www.amensolution.com) to find out which of your brain systems might need help and what specific supplements might be of benefit to you.

Take the 24/7 Brain Gym Assessment on Brain Health—Also on www.amensolution.com, you will find an individualized set of exercises in the form of fun games to optimize your brain. You can join for just a dollar for two weeks, and stay longer if you like.

Know Your Important Numbers—Write them down where you can see them and work to optimize them. If you don't have all of the test results I recommend, ask your health care provider to order the following lab studies. If he or she will not order them, consider seeing someone who will. You want to be the leader of your health team. You can also order these tests yourself at websites such as SaveOnLabs.com.

4

BALANCE YOUR HORMONES TO BOOST THE FEMALE BRAIN

PART ONE: BALANCE ESTROGEN, PROGESTERONE, AND TESTOSTERONE
PART TWO: BALANCE THYROID, CORTISOL, DHEA, AND INSULIN

Optimizing your major hormones is the fourth step to unleashing the power of the female brain.
Well, I knew something was wrong with me when my usual charming self thought it okay to flip someone off who irritated me on the freeway—thank goodness I don't live in LA or NYC, I'd probably be dead!"

—ONE OF MY PATIENTS WHILE EXPERIENCING PMS

"I just don't feel right."
"I have brain fog."
"My memory is worse than ever."
"I hurt all over."
"I can't sleep."

"I have no interest in sex."

"I just yelled at my teenage daughter for no reason. I hate myself."

"I feel like I am going to crawl out of my skin."

"I am hungrier than ever."

These are common complaints I hear from my female patients, and they all can be hormone-related. Knowing how to test, balance, and optimize your hormones is critical to unleashing the power of your female brain.

Of course, hormonal issues don't just apply to females. Just look at any teenage boy. And scientists are now talking about a male midlife change—andropause. But having five sisters, three daughters, and a teenage granddaughter, I know that male swings are nothing like the wild ride of hormones that women face. For many men, levels of the male sex hormone testosterone peak at around age eighteen and then go into a long, steady slide through old age. For a woman, hormonal changes often feel like a roller coaster that goes through peaks, valleys, quick turns, and abrupt stops.

Females enter puberty with a shock. Probably every woman remembers her first menses. And that monthly reminder persists for years, driven by a hormonal cycle that can affect your feelings and thought patterns and give you acne to boot. Then there's the tsunami of hormones that comes with pregnancy, childbirth, and postpartum changes. Finally, after years of hormonal cycling, you face the perfect storm of perimenopause and menopause with too many hormones here, not enough hormones there, and all of it out of whack.

So what can you do?

It turns out there's a lot you can do. New research and clinical work now offers workable solutions to women who are ready to take back control of their hormones and their lives.

YOUR BRAIN IS RUN BY HORMONES

The human body is an amazing assortment of organ systems. When everything works together, your body plays like a precisely tuned orchestra where your brain, ovaries, adrenal glands, pancreas, and thyroid do what they're supposed to at the right time. Your brain gets active or stays quiet as needed. Your organs play a sweet, steady note together, and your sense of well-being reflects the harmony within. You feel happy and energetic. You sleep well and have good digestion. Your stress is under control. There are no sour notes. Life is beautiful.

But for that harmony to exist, all the different parts of the orchestra have to communicate with each other so they know when they need to play loud, soft, or stop playing altogether. And that's where your hormones come in. Hormones are chemical messengers produced by certain organs that travel through the bloodstream, keeping cells and other organs informed of what's going on so everyone can come in on cue.

Your hormones are a delicate system that can be affected by many factors, both inside and outside your body. Problems start when hormones fall into a state of imbalance. Maybe the thyroid produces too much hormone, or too little, and everything else goes haywire. And women are more likely than men to have these problems.

Fortunately, our knowledge of hormones and how to put them back into balance is growing. You have at your disposal many tools you can use to work with the challenges your hormones put you through so you can put yourself back in control.

But we have to start where we are, so let's look at what happens when things are not working right.

There are two main issues women experience with hormone imbalances: uncomfortable symptoms that can begin to change how you think, feel, and act, affecting your quality of life, and an increased risk of illnesses, such as depression, Alzheimer's disease, heart disease, osteoporosis, diabetes, and certain cancers.

Do any of the following scenarios sound like you?

You've been gaining weight and you don't know why. You suspect it's because of the bag of chips and salsa you eat every night with a couple of glasses of wine, but you don't understand where these cravings are coming from and why you can't stop yourself from giving in to them.

Or maybe you feel depressed, anxious, or irritable for no apparent reason. It's tempting to blame your disrespectful kids or your unresponsive husband or your annoying mother-in-law. But are they really the cause? Why do they become especially irksome during certain times of the month?

Or do you wake up in the middle of the night, wracked with worry and plagued by thoughts that are going so fast they jam up against each other? Your husband is happily snoring away right next to you. Why isn't he as obsessed over the broken water heater as you are?

There is a very strong mutual influence between hormones and the brain. The brain produces signals that trigger hormones and hormones from other parts of the body also influence the brain. For example, when thyroid activity is low, brain activity is typically low as well. That's why a low thyroid often goes along with depression, irritability, and brain fog. Balanced hormones are critical to your brain's well-being.

MEET THE CAST OF CHARACTERS

There are hundreds of hormones in the body that affect the brain. To keep it practical, I am going to show you how to optimize seven of your most important hormones:

- Estrogen
- Progesterone

- Testosterone
- Thyroid
- Cortisol
- DHEA
- Insulin

Owing to the importance and complexity of the topic I have divided Chapter 4 into two parts.

PART ONE: BALANCE ESTROGEN, PROGESTERONE, AND TESTOSTERONE

When you have a deficiency of progesterone and an imbalance of hormones, it literally feels like the "decision part" of your brain has been taken away from you. Women describe feeling like they are watching themselves handle situations with anger and frustration, as if they were someone else.

—TAMI MERAGLIA, M.D.,
INTEGRATIVE MEDICINE PHYSICIAN

ESTROGEN AND PROGESTERONE: THE FEMALE SEX HORMONES

Estrogen

Estrogen helps you think clearly. Progesterone helps you relax.

Two of the major hormones that drive your menstrual cycle are estrogen and progesterone. They are much more than just reproductive hormones. They actually affect many systems in the body, including bones, cardiovascular system, reproductive system, and your brain. And they are not just found in women. They are also found in men, only in much smaller amounts, unless the males are obese or have other estrogen-producing conditions.

A woman's menstrual cycle reflects the natural rising and falling of estrogen and progesterone during a typical twenty-eight-day cycle. When everything works correctly, estrogen rises and falls twice during that time frame, in a gentle rolling motion, while progesterone rises and falls once. The chart below shows the cycle of *estradiol,* one of the key forms of estrogen, and progesterone. More about the different forms of estrogen in a bit.

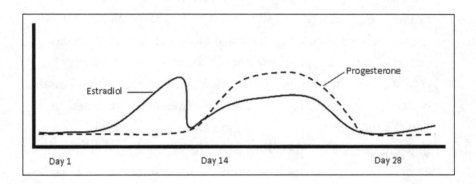

Healthy levels of estrogen help you feel good. Too much estrogen can make you feel as anxious and irritable as a wet cat. Estrogen withdrawal makes you feel depressed and confused. It's the rise and drop in estrogen that drastically affects your mood, and the more erratic your particular fluctuation is, the more upset it can make you. These problems become worse during perimenopause and menopause, when estrogen levels wane.

There are three different kinds of estrogen: *estrone, estradiol,* and *estriol.* According to my friend and colleague Dr. James LaValle, author of the *Metabolic Code,* estrone is the estrogen to worry about. Estrone can make you more prone to cancer.

Your liver, gut, and adrenal health determine what types of hormones are made. Depending on how you take care of your body, you can push your body to make healthy or unhealthy estrogens, which is why getting healthy is critical to all of your body's systems, including your brain. As women age, their estradiol and estriol levels go down, and their estrone levels increase.

Estrone—Estrone is the main estrogen made by women after menopause and is implicated in breast and uterine cancer. Before menopause, women make all three estrogens and progesterone. The majority of estrone is made in the liver, adrenal glands, and fat tissue. After menopause, the levels of estradiol, estriol, and progesterone drop drastically, and their health protective effects are lost. It's not surprising that the majority of breast cancer cases occur in postmenopausal women. Obese women are at higher risk. Alcohol consumption also increases estrone, which could be the reason there is an association between alcohol intake and breast cancer. Estrone production is also increased with excess sugar, the antacid cimetidine (sold under the brand name Tagamet), birth control pills, hypothyroidism, smoking, and pesticide exposure.

Estradiol—Estradiol is the strongest estrogen; it helps you think clearly. It is produced in the ovaries and has many protective effects, including maintaining bone density, improving growth hormone production and cardiovascular function, keeping your blood from getting "sticky," supporting cognitive function and mood, assisting in growth hormone release, and improving your lipid profile. Too much estradiol can be associated with estrogen-related cancers, but deficiencies can lead to osteoporosis, heart disease, dementia, and other diseases of aging. Estradiol keeps you looking and feeling young and vibrant. It also provides antiaging protection for the skin. And it even helps prevent weight gain. Researchers at Yale University have found that estradiol suppresses appetite using the same pathways in the brain as leptin, which is one of the hormones that regulate appetite. In perimenopause and menopause, estradiol begins to decrease, which might be one of the reasons that menopausal women find it so difficult to control their weight. They're just hungry all the time.

Estriol—Estriol is the weakest of the three estrogens and has a protective role in breast tissue. It is believed to protect vaginal tissue too. Estriol helps to reduce hot flashes in women, protects the urinary tract, and plays a role in retention of bone density. It can help increase "good" HDL and decrease "bad" LDL cholesterol. One compelling study showed that taking estriol can reverse brain lesions in women with multiple sclerosis.

Estrogen is particularly needed in women to make serotonin function at its best in the brain. Serotonin is one of the brain's feel good hormones. With no estrogen, your mood can change to anxious and depressed. Cognitive function, such as critical thinking and short-term memory, is also eroded with the loss of estrogen production.

Below is a list of symptoms related to low and high estrogen levels:

Low Estrogen
    Weight gain
    Bladder incontinence and infection
    Mood changes/depression
    Insomnia
    Low libido
    Heart palpitations
    Osteoporosis
    Painful intercourse

Foggy-headedness

Irritability

Fatigue

Weepiness

Hot flashes

Pain

Excess Estrogen

Puffiness

Heavy bleeding

Fibrocystic breasts

Low libido

Cravings for carbohydrates

Weight gain around the hips

Vaginal or oral yeast (thrush)

Mood swings / easy to tear

Tender breasts

Headaches or migraines

In a young, healthy woman, the estrogen ratio generally averages as follows: 60–80 percent estriol, 10–20 percent estradiol, and 10–20 percent estrone. While these levels vary from one individual to another, the goal of bioidentical hormone restoration therapy (BHRT), discussed later, is to re-create a more natural balance in the levels of estrogen and in combination with all the other sex hormones.

Estrogens convert into several metabolites. Estrone, for example, may convert into three different forms:

- 2-hydroxyestrone, protective against cancer
- 4-hydroxyestrone, promotes cancer
- 16-alpha-hydroxyestrone, promotes cancer

2-hydroxyestrone is considered a "good estrogen" metabolite, whereas 4-hydroxyestrone and 16-alpha-hydroxyestrone have been associated with the development of certain types of cancer, like breast and ovarian. These "bad estrogens" are also associated with uterine fibroids, ovarian cysts, and fibrocystic breasts.

The main areas for estrogen breakdown are the liver and gastrointestinal tract. *Diets high in refined sugar and low in fiber feed the unfriendly bacteria in the intestines, causing them to disrupt estrogen metabolism.* One of the by-products of the unfriendly "bugs" in the intestines is that the estrogen metabolites can't be excreted and they build up in your tissues over time, causing trouble.

The relationship between 2-hydroxyestrone (good estrogen) and 16-alpha-hydroxyestrone (bad estrogen) is expressed as the 2:16 ratio. The higher the ratio, the better. The minimum acceptable number ratio is 2 and ideally it is greater than 4. Lower ratios are associated with breast and ovarian cancers. You can easily be tested for this ratio with a simple in-home urine test available online.

Dietary Changes to Improve the 2:16 Ratio

There are great foods that can help improve the conversion of estrogen into good metabolites and away from the bad ones. These foods include *insoluble dietary fibers*, such as lignin found in green beans, peas, carrots, seeds, and Brazil nuts. The reason that dietary fiber, especially lignin, is so beneficial is that it can bind harmful estrogens in the digestive tract, so they can be excreted in the feces instead of being reabsorbed. Dietary fiber also improves the composition of intestinal bacteria so that harmful estrogen metabolites can be excreted from the body. It also decreases the conversion of testosterone into estrogens, maintaining a healthy testosterone level.

Sugar and simple carbohydrates cause unfriendly flora to grow in the gastrointestinal tract and disrupt estrogen metabolism. These foods also raise blood sugar and insulin levels, resulting in adverse influences in sex hormone balance. Too many simple carbohydrates have been associated with postmenopausal breast cancer risk among overweight women and women with a large waist circumference.

Avoid animal protein that has been raised with hormones or antibiotics whenever possible. Europe won't accept hormone-laden U.S. beef because of the health risks. Look for grass-fed, hormone-free, antibiotic-free organic beef and chicken, which is richer in omega-3 fatty acids and will therefore act to reduce inflammation and help your hormone receptors to function properly. Also, eat organic vegetables, fruits, nuts, seeds, beans, and grains.

Pesticides are known to cause hormonal imbalances and some pesticides have been shown to act as "endocrine (hormone) disrupters," interfering with the body's natural hormone systems and causing an array of health problems. While the Environmental Protection Agency began looking at this issue in 1999, little change has yet occurred in the marketplace, and women are well served to educate themselves on this important issue. (I'll discuss this more later in this chapter.)

Lifestyle Changes to Improve the 2:16 Ratio

Your lifestyle may expose you to environmental estrogens that can disrupt your body's natural balance or interfere with proper therapy. Here are some tips from Dr. LaValle to reduce your exposure:

1. Limit drinking out of plastic containers, and when you do, drink only from containers that are free of bisphenol A, better known as BPA.
2. Do not microwave food in plastic containers or covered in plastic.
3. Avoid using personal care items such as face creams, cosmetics, shampoos, tampons, and toiletries that contain environmental estrogens and particularly phthalates. Phthalates are

synthetic substances found in many plastics. They have estrogenic properties and are banned as a toxic substance in Europe.

Dietary Supplements to Improve Estrogen Metabolism

Diindolylmethane (DIM)—This is a phytochemical found in cruciferous vegetables like broccoli and cauliflower. It shifts estrogen metabolism to favor the friendly or harmless estrogen metabolites. DIM can significantly increase the urinary excretion of the "bad" estrogens in as little as four weeks. The typical dose of DIM is 75–300 mg per day.

Omega-3 Fatty Acids (fish oils)—These contain eicosapentaenoic acid (EPA), which has been reported in laboratory studies to help control estrogen metabolism and decrease the risk of breast cancer. Eating grass-fed organic beef also supplies these fats. I typically recommend 2,000 mg a day.

Calcium d-glucarate—This natural compound is found in fruits and vegetables like apples, Brussels sprouts, broccoli, and cabbage. Calcium d-glucarate inhibits the enzyme that contributes to breast, prostate, and colon cancers. It also reduces reabsorbed estrogen from the digestive tract. The dose for calcium d-glucarate is typically 500–1,500 mg per day.

Probiotics—These help maintain healthy intestinal flora and healthy estrogen levels. Make sure you get human-strain probiotics that have live cultures. Consider taking 10–60 billion units per day.

Plant Phytoestrogens—These plant-based compounds have healthy estrogen-like activity and have been found helpful for a variety of conditions, including menopausal symptoms, PMS, and endometriosis. Phytoestrogens can be found in soy, kudzu, red clover, and pomegranate. Resveratrol is a bioflavonoid antioxidant that occurs naturally in grapes and red wine and has been reported to inhibit breast cancer cell growth in laboratory studies.

Black cohosh is an herb that's been used for centuries by Native Americans for hormonal balance in women. Over the last thirty years, European physicians helping women through menopausal transition have used it extensively. In human studies, black cohosh has been found to decrease hot flashes associated with menopause. Unlike conventional estrogen effects on individuals predisposed to breast cancer, black cohosh has been shown in laboratory studies to inhibit cancer cells. Most studies used doses of 20 to 80 mg twice daily, providing 4–8 mg triterpene glycosides for up to six months.

> **Melatonin**—This hormone is produced in the pineal gland that, among other functions, helps sleep. Melatonin levels decline with age and may lead to the sleep disturbances common during menopause. Melatonin has been shown in laboratory studies to inhibit the growth of breast cancer cells. Melatonin acts as an anti-inflammatory and antioxidant in the brain and other tissues like the intestine. Studies show that low melatonin levels increase breast cancer risk in women. So if you are having trouble sleeping consider 3–6 mg of melatonin before bed. It may boost your immune system and help you sleep.

Estrogen and Pain

A study in the *Journal of Neuroscience* tested pain sensitivity in women at different times during their menstrual cycle—first during their period when estradiol is at its lowest and then when their estradiol levels were at their highest. The women in the study were subjected to a controlled amount of pain and asked to rate the level of their discomfort. At low levels of estradiol, the women reported feeling much more pain than when the hormone was at its highest. The implication is that when your estrogen levels are low, such as during menopause or during the premenstrual or menstrual phase of your cycle, you are likely to feel pain more acutely, which is also likely true for emotional pain. Just one more reason a smart man is especially sensitive at this time!

Progesterone

Progesterone can support GABA (gama-aminobutyric acid; a major calming neurotransmitter in the brain) and the myelin sheath—it is much more than a sex hormone.

The other major hormonal player in your cycle is progesterone. It helps to prepare the uterus for implantation with a healthy fertilized egg and supports pregnancy. If no implantation occurs, progesterone levels drop, and another cycle begins.

Progesterone receptors are highly concentrated in the brain. Progesterone can support GABA, the brain's relaxation neurotransmitter, acts to protect your nerve cells, and supports the myelin sheath that covers neurons. I like to think of progesterone as the "feel-good hormone." It makes you feel calm and peaceful and encourages sleep. It's like nature's Valium, but better, because instead of making your brain fuzzy, it sharpens your thinking. It has also been shown to help with brain injuries by reducing inflammation and counteracting damage. It is so much more than a sex hormone.

Progesterone increases during pregnancy, which is why many pregnant women often feel great. Some women with hormonal issues, in fact, feel so much better during pregnancy that they will deliberately get pregnant over and over again just trying to feel normal. Other than during pregnancy, it's rare to see women with too much progesterone. However, women who are given too much progesterone (like taking too much Valium) can get depressed and feel as they would during the first few weeks of pregnancy, with morning sickness, sleepiness, and a dull backache.

Progesterone is low for the first two weeks of the menstrual cycle. Then it follows a rolling-hill pattern during the second half of the cycle, rising and falling along with estrogen. A drop in progesterone means the loss of the feel-good hormone. Calmness gives way to anxiety and irritability. Sleep is disturbed. Things get a bit fuzzy. Along with estrogen, progesterone plummets right before menstruation starts, and for some women, that's when the bottom falls out. Her hormonal mainstays have all fallen away. Here are some common symptoms:

Low Progesterone
>   Anxiety/Depression
>   Trouble sleeping
>   Fibrocystic breasts
>   PMS
>   Premenstrual headaches
>   Postpartum depression
>   Bone loss

Progesterone can fluctuate greatly in women who are in their late thirties and forties, making them feel anxious and out of sorts. Often progesterone cream can be very helpful under the care of an experienced health care provider.

Progesterone production can decrease with low levels of thyroid hormone, the use of antidepressants, chronic stress, deficiencies in the vitamins A, B_6, C, or zinc, and a diet high in refined sugar. Chasteberry has been found to help support healthy progesterone levels. It can also be taken to reduce the symptoms of PMS and endometriosis (20–40 mg a day).

PMS: THE MONTHLY CYCLE CAN BE MURDER

I know that PMS is real. With all the estrogen in my world, I've experienced it firsthand. One of my sisters or daughters can think I walk on water one week and then want to throw rocks at me the next. But seeing PMS show up on a brain scan really clinched it for me. My patients have proved to me that PMS is more than just a hormone issue. It's actually a brain disorder, and Jesse was one of the women to show me what it looks like. I first saw Jesse after she split from her husband. During a fight, she pulled knife on him and told him not to go to sleep. He left her that evening. It turned out that Jesse had long-standing temper issues that paralleled her menstrual cycle. Regularly in the week before her period started, she became moody, anxious, and aggressive. And she aggravated the problem by drinking a lot. The incident with the knife had occurred at precisely this point in her cycle.

When Jesse came to see me, I knew it would be helpful to find out what was going on in her brain. I scanned her during the worst part of her cycle, and then again, two weeks later, when she usually felt her best. The results were striking. The two sets of scans didn't even look like they came from the same person. During the worst time of Jesse's cycle, the "worry" region of her brain was overactive, which caused her to become fixated on things, and the judgment and impulse control part of her brain was underactive. The alcohol likely further dropped her ability to control her behavior. That's why she was so distraught with her husband and why grabbing the knife seemed like a good idea. During the best time of her cycle, Jesse's brain was much more balanced. The answer to this woman's problem was not just anger-management therapy. It was to get her hormonal fluctuations under control.

During the days prior to starting your period, estrogen and

progesterone levels hit rock bottom. On scans, I see the worry center of the brain (the anterior cingulate gyrus) start to fire up; as a result, women can get stuck on negative thoughts or give in to behaviors they think will make them feel better, such as reaching for wine or cookies. This makes sense, because the anterior cingulate is the part of your brain that helps you shift attention, be flexible, and go with the flow.

The anterior cingulate fires up as the end result of a series of events. First estrogen falls. As it does, serotonin, the feel-good neurotransmitter, also falls. The deficiency in serotonin causes the anterior cingulate gyrus to fire up. To make things worse, just about this time the PFC tends to quiet down, which is why women may have a hard time focusing and controlling impulses. So we see emotional difficulties, intensified feelings of sadness, and disturbed sleep.

This is hard enough to deal with on a monthly basis. But by the time you hit your later thirties, your body is less efficient at producing progesterone. And in your forties, your progesterone curve stops creating that nice hill and looks more like a bump. Research shows that progesterone levels start to decrease eight years before a woman goes into menopause, and this is when progesterone withdrawal symptoms can become more pronounced. Memory declines and it's hard to concentrate. You experience mood swings. Your brain has lost its natural sleeping pill and antianxiety hormone. This can lead to marital problems and sometimes even addictions.

The Myriad PMS Symptoms

- Acne
- Alcohol sensitivity
- Anger
- Anxiety
- Appetite changes
- Bloating
- Breast tenderness

Jesse's SPECT Scans

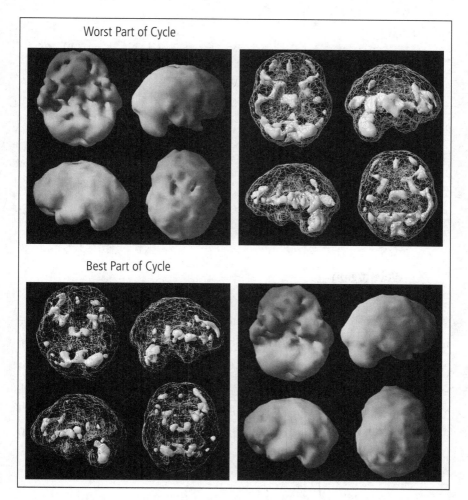

Worst Part of Cycle

Best Part of Cycle

- Clumsiness
- Confusion
- Constipation
- Cramps
- Cravings for sweet or salty foods
- Crying spells
- Decreased sex drive

- Depression
- Distractibility
- Fatigue
- Forgetful
- Headaches and possible migraines
- Herpes outbreaks
- Impulsivity
- Insomnia
- Irritability
- Mood swings
- Panic attacks
- Suspiciousness
- Tearfulness
- Weight gain

PMS symptoms can be precipitated by oral contraceptives, pregnancies, miscarriages, abortions, tubal ligations, partial hysterectomies, aging, and low magnesium levels and exacerbated by low blood sugar, caffeine, poor diet, and skipping meals. Complicating matters, these symptoms are frequently misdiagnosed as psychiatric disorders, such as anxiety, depression, panic attacks, agoraphobia, eating disorders, and personality disorders.

Help for PMS—Low progesterone is often one of the culprits of PMS symptoms. Progesterone cream used during the last week of a woman's cycle is often helpful. I also recommend a combination of supplements to balance the brain, especially 400–500 mg calcium citrate twice a day, 200–300 mg chelated magnesium twice a day, vitamin A, B complex with 50 mg B_6, and 500 mg evening primrose oil twice a day. I also suggest 50–100 mg 5-HTP (5-hydroxytryptophan) twice a day to help to boost serotonin and decrease anxiety and worry. If focus is a problem, try green tea or

500 mg L-tyrosine two to three times a day. Chasteberry, 20–40 mg a day, can also help for PMS symptoms of especially breast pain or tenderness, swelling, constipation, irritability, depressed mood or mood alterations, anger, and headache in some women. Boost exercise the last week of your cycle, and hold the sugar and alcohol.

TESTOSTERONE

Most people think of testosterone as the male hormone. It's a shot of testosterone during a critical time of fetal development that creates the male brain. And another shot of this hormone during puberty leads to the deepening voice, facial hair, and many of the other features we associate with "maleness." But females have testosterone too (just as males have some estrogen), and testosterone can do wonderful things for a woman. It helps protect her nervous system and wards off cognitive impairment, depression, and Alzheimer's disease. It also seems to protect cells from inflammation, which some researchers believe is why men are less susceptible to inflammatory diseases like rheumatoid arthritis, psoriasis, and asthma than are women, and even why they suffer less from depression. Men who have low testosterone are more likely to suffer from chronic pain, which is more common in women.

As many as 20 percent of women are low in testosterone and therefore have decreased sensitivity to sexual pleasure coupled with a low sex drive. Combine that with poor memory and depression, and these hormonal fluctuations can mean big trouble in a woman's life: the quality of her engagement in relationships, her ability to be emotionally and physically intimate with a partner, her enjoyment of sex, and her effectiveness in her personal and professional work.

Keeping the right level of testosterone is important for your health and well-being. Too much can cause major health problems, but too little is associated with depression, poor memory, and low libido. This is not a good recipe for intimate relationships. Many couples fall in love when their hormones are balanced or at their highest levels. When testosterone levels drop, so does a woman's interest in sex as well as her sensitivity to sexual pleasure (testosterone affects the sensitivity of the nipples and clitoris), which can cause serious relationship problems.

Low Testosterone Levels?

Besides increased libido, there are other benefits related to testosterone replacement for women, including retention of muscle mass and bone density, improved mood, and reduced cardiovascular risks. Levels of testosterone in the blood should be checked to see if they are low before using any type of bioidentical testosterone or even dietary supplements, such as DHEA (I'll discuss DHEA in the next part of this chapter), which can raise testosterone levels.

Before you let your doctor give you testosterone shots or pills, try to boost it naturally by dramatically decreasing or even eliminating sugar, wheat, and processed foods from your diet. A sugar burst has been found to lower testosterone levels by up to 25 percent.

If you and your sweetheart share the cheesecake at the restaurant, no one is likely to get "dessert" when you get home!

Another way to naturally boost your testosterone level is to start a weight-training program. Building muscle helps your body increase its testosterone levels. The supplements DHEA and zinc can also help. Zinc is necessary to maintain normal testosterone levels. Inadequate zinc levels prevent the pituitary gland from releasing hormones that stimulate testosterone production. Zinc also inhibits the enzyme that converts testosterone into estrogen. If these measures don't work, you may need testosterone replacement.

Get your testosterone level checked and start with natural ways to normalize it when it is low.

What Steals Your Testosterone Levels
- Abdominal fat
- Stress
- Excess sugar, processed foods, and insulin
- Zinc deficiency
- Alcohol

Polycystic Ovary Syndrome

Too much testosterone is often associated with polycystic ovary syndrome (PCOS) in which multiple cysts appear in the ovaries. It is associated with irregular periods, acne, excessive facial and body hair, and sometimes aggression. It has been associated with serious health problems such as obesity, high cholesterol, high blood pressure, diabetes, infertility, and hypersexuality, which makes women more vulnerable to affairs. The diagnosis of PCOS is often suspected in women who are heavyset (abdominal obesity) and prediabetic and who have facial hair, balding, interstitial cystitis, irritable bowel syndrome, and high inflammatory markers. Their lab work often shows high levels of dihydrotestosterone (DHT), high blood sugar levels, low progesterone levels relative to estrogen, and a high level of follicle-stimulating hormone (FSH).

One of the best tests to diagnose PCOS is an ultrasound of the ovaries, where you can see multiple cysts on each ovary.

Sometimes PCOS Can Fool You—None of the many physicians my wife saw ever mentioned the possibility of PCOS to her, despite her complaining of irregular periods. She just didn't look like the typical female with PCOS. Tana is extremely fit and has gorgeous, thick red hair. At about thirty-eight years of age, Tana went off birth control pills and she soon realized that something odd was going on. Her face started breaking out and her menstrual cycles became very irregular. Although it seemed she was too young, she thought she might be going through peri-menopause. It seemed best to see her doctor right away to determine what was going on—and the results were shocking. Tana was dismayed to learn that her cholesterol and triglycerides were high and that she was prediabetic. How was that possible? Tana is 5 foot 6 inches, weighs 121 pounds, and has about 15 percent body fat. She works out like a nut and eats all the right foods. "That's crazy," she thought. "I'm the healthiest person I know."

We were both very concerned, and that's when a friend introduced us to an integrative gynecologist who did an ultrasound on Tana's ovaries and found they both contained dozens of cysts. She diagnosed Tana with PCOS. How would her doctor have known about Tana's ovaries unless she looked at them? PCOS was also linked to Tana's other symptoms, including irregular menstrual cycles, skin breakouts, high cholesterol, and insulin resistance. We were lucky that we found a physician smart enough to check for this since Tana doesn't fit the typical physical profile of a woman with PCOS.

Tana's treatment was simple, but it led to dramatic changes. She was prescribed glucophage, a medication used to balance insulin, and that, in turn, reduces testosterone levels. In addition, she was given a bioidentical progesterone cream, saw palmetto to drive down her high levels of DHT, and a comprehensive stress-reduction program. Within a few months, Tana's cholesterol dropped 50 points, her insulin levels normalized, her skin cleared up, and her cycle became regular. She was also less anxious and wanted to cuddle more. "Good for me," I thought.

THE PILL: WHAT YOU NEED TO KNOW

Tens of millions of women take hormones daily in the form of oral contraceptive pills (OCPs). In the United States alone, forty-three million women of child-bearing age do not want to become pregnant, and of those, 28 percent take OCPs.

Over the years, OCPs have been both hailed as the best thing that ever happened to the modern woman and vilified as a hidden health threat. Certainly it has given women considerable control over their destinies by allowing them to delay having children, limit the size of their families, and arrange the timing of their pregnancies. But there is also evidence that OCPs are not completely benign. It has been shown to cause problems with blood pressure and blood clots and to increase the incidence of strokes, especially in women who smoke or who have a history of migraine headaches. Smoking while on OCPs can be extremely dangerous.

Typically, birth control pills are formulated with estrogen and progestin (a synthetic form of progesterone). The estrogen is usually in synthetic form as well. This combination functions by preventing ovulation. Nothing happens in a vacuum, though, and this mix of hormones has additional effects on the body. If you are on OCPs you should be aware of these effects so you can take steps to counter them if necessary.

For one thing, oral contraceptives deplete some of the essential vitamins and minerals and can lead to deficiencies. If you are taking birth control pills, you should be supplementing your diet with B vitamins (folate, B_6, and B_{12}), and vitamin E. You should also be looking for signs of a magnesium deficiency, which can lead to a variety of symptoms:

- Anxiety, nervousness, and insomnia
- Depression, migraines, and low energy
- Muscle cramps and spasms
- Heart arrhythmias and palpitations
- Constipation
- Blood sugar dysregulation
- Hypertension

If you find yourself suffering from symptoms like these, you can take a magnesium supplement. The usual dose is 300–800 mg elemental magnesium daily. A good way to judge the dosage is to achieve a soft stool without taking it to the point of diarrhea. There are a variety of magnesium salts to choose from. The right one for you is based on your specific needs:

- Magnesium malate is good for fibromyalgia, leg cramps, and workout issues such as lactic acid buildup.
- Magnesium taurate helps with anxiety and arrhythmias.
- Magnesium glycinate has the best absorption.
- Magnesium citrate is inexpensive, if cost is an issue.
- Magnesium carbonate and magnesium oxide are not the best choices, as they do not absorb well.

Another symptom reported by 16–56 percent of women on OCPs is bouts of depression. Scientists have argued for years over the role of the pill in causing depression. In a recent review of the literature, the authors cited the inconsistent use of the term *depression* and the varied formulations of the birth control pills taken as making it difficult to draw firm conclusions. However, there have been studies with clear results. For example, a study by Jayashri Kulkarni of Monash University in Australia found that women who were on OCPs were almost twice as likely to be depressed as the women who were not on the pill. The nonusers had a depression score of 9.8, whereas women who were on the pill had a depression score of 17.6. One reason for this effect may be that progestin acts as natural progesterone does to lower brain serotonin, an important neurotransmitter for the regulation of mood. Another contributing factor may be an increase in copper levels in women on OCPs.

As with any drug you take, the effects may be far-reaching. Be aware of what's happening in your body. As we have seen, a woman's hormones significantly affect her mood and her body chemistry. Adding birth control pills into the mix is sure to shake things up. Be prepared to take supplements to counteract any negative effects, and if you start feeling symptoms of depression that interfere with your life, discuss it with your doctor.

THE BEGINNING OF A NEW PHASE: PERIMENOPAUSE

By the time you reach your thirties or forties, your hormones start undergoing another change. Your body is preparing itself to go out of the baby-making business and that means shuffling around the hormone balance once more.

It doesn't all happen overnight. For eight to ten years before entering menopause (when your menstrual cycle ends completely), you will go through a period of adjustment known as perimenopause. Most women don't think about being in perimenopause until their estrogen levels have fallen to a point where they get hit with hot flashes and night sweats, the most common symptoms. But by the time you are having hot flashes, you've probably been going through perimenopause for up to ten years.

These years of adjustment can be a difficult time. Your hormone system doesn't work as efficiently as it did, and the once (relatively) gentle ups and downs in your hormone levels give way to estrogen spikes followed by a crash right before your period begins. The result can be severe PMS symptoms, even if you've never had them before. When estrogen levels decline during the menstrual cycle, perimenopause, or menopause, you also have more trouble with your short-term memory and are more likely to have crying spells and depression. You may find yourself forgetting where you put your keys or what you came to the grocery store to pick up. Low levels of estrogen can also make you more sensitive to pain. All these symptoms are exaggerated with the more erratic hormonal shifts in perimenopause. The seesaw effect of going from estrogen dominance to estrogen withdrawal becomes more pronounced. It isn't fun for you (or those around you), and it can make you feel as though you are literally losing your mind.

Your awareness of what's going on can help you weather the hormonal storms during this time and even thrive. These are the years when you can make tremendous strides in your personal growth, deepen your relationships, and make advancements in your career. You don't want hormonal shifts to interfere with reaching your full potential. To help you stay on top of the situation, it is a good idea to get your hormone levels checked when you are about thirty-five years old so you have a baseline. Then get them checked every two to three years. This is much better than waiting—as many women we see in our clinic have done—until you are ten years into the process, have already put on an extra 35 pounds, and are on antidepressant and antianxiety medications. Intervening earlier in the process can help you avoid a lot of problems.

Maintaining a brain-healthy lifestyle will improve your hormonal balance all around. Committing to exercise, meditation, and the proper diet while avoiding nicotine, too much alcohol and caffeine, and unhealthy foods, will make things go much more smoothly. If you and your doctor decide you could use more help in balancing your hormones, BHRT is available in the form of creams, pills, and vaginal inserts (more on BHRT on p. 000). If you're having hot flashes, these can be effectively treated with a combination of estradiol and estriol. You can also find natural treatments in the form of supplements, such as B vitamins, fish oil, evening primrose oil, and flaxseed oil.

IT'S NOT YOUR GRANDMOTHER'S MENOPAUSE

Menopause just isn't what it used to be. When I think of my grandmother Marcella, my father's mother, whom I adored, she was already an old woman in her fifties and sixties. She often appeared tired and out of breath, was overweight, and wore simple clothes. She died at age sixty-two. In contrast, my mother, at eighty-one, remains vibrant and active. She still plays golf; dresses in a stylish way; and is often found at the mall with one of my sisters, daughters, or nieces. For many women in menopause, they are at the peak of their careers and social life.

If you're going through menopause now, you realize that it's not the end of anything vital to who you really are. If anything, it's an opportunity for new freedom in the many decades of life ahead. But with the physical changes in menopause, there are still some challenges to be faced. Your understanding of what's going on can help you make these the best years of your life.

Menopause is the permanent end of your menstrual cycle. Technically it is the one-year mark after your last period. After that point you are said to be postmenopausal. Of course, this is a rather arbitrary cut-off point and you may continue to experience many of the symptoms you had during perimenopause. Plus, since your estrogen and progesterone have probably fallen to very low levels, you can no longer benefit from their protective qualities. You're now more vulnerable to conditions such as heart disease, stroke, and Alzheimer's disease, and your bones may also be thinning. You may struggle with cognitive effects as well. Because menopause often comes with lower overall brain activity, it can be associated with depression, anxiety, insomnia, weight gain, and problems with concentration and memory.

It is even more critical during this time to take brain health seriously, as the reserve in your brain has declined.

When I was preparing for my last public television show, I called up my mother and asked her to get an audience for me so I could practice the script. Afterward, one of her sixty-year-old friends commented that at her age she didn't want to have to worry anymore about what she eats or exercising. If that is your attitude too, you'll just want to make sure you're okay with the consequences of having an older brain: less energy, brain fog, depression, and more bad decisions. As we age, we have less room for error. To be better, you have to be constantly vigilant for your health and not let others steal it.

We now have proof that the sex hormones are in fact critical for brain health. Studies of women who have complete hysterectomies, in which their ovaries are removed, show that without hormone replacement they have double the risk for Alzheimer's disease. Recently, researchers studied the brain scans of a group of women who were on and off hormone replacement. Over a period of two years, the woman who did not take hormone replacement showed decreased activity in an area of the brain called the posterior cingulate gyrus. This finding is especially significant because that is one of the first areas in the brain that dies in Alzheimer's disease. The women who were taking hormone replacement showed no reduced activity in that area of the brain.

BIOIDENTICAL HORMONE REPLACEMENT THERAPY—FOR BRAIN AND BODY

Hormones are derived from other hormones in a kind of family tree that is illustrated below. The first hormone in the series is cholesterol. We've all heard lots of bad things about cholesterol, but the fact is, it isn't the enemy. Yes, when it's too high, cholesterol is associated with heart disease. But when it's too low, it can be associated with homicide, suicide, and severe depression. You need cholesterol in your brain and your body. About 60 percent of the solid weight of your brain is fat. Your brain and your body need healthy cholesterol levels to function optimally.

From cholesterol, your body next makes a "mother" hormone called pregnenolone from which a host of others hormones are derived. Your doctor can influence your hormonal balance at any point in the tree depending on your individual needs. For example, if you take pregnenolone, your body can choose on its own which hormones are deficient and will make what it needs. Or your doctor may decide to prescribe testosterone, progesterone, or one of the estrogens. With our growing understanding of how hormones interact and the availability of safer medications, including bioidentical hormones and natural options, we can now pinpoint treatments that can help you function at your best.

HORMONAL CASCADE

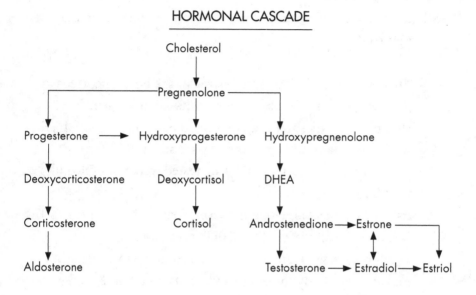

Before we discuss BHRT, it is important to always remember that simply replacing any hormones without improving the way you process and utilize them can be a very problematic. To maximize the benefits of BHRT, you need to make the brain-healthy changes in your life. Eating healthier, taking supplements where needed, getting more sleep, and exercising will have a synergistic effect.

Diminishing sex hormones during perimenopause and menopause have been shown to cause a number of disturbing symptoms. In the past, scientists worked on ways to replace those hormones with therapeutic doses of natural or synthetic hormones. Many women found relief, and it looked as though hormone replacement therapy (HRT) would be the wave of the future. Then certain health problems began to crop up. In 2002, the World Health Initiative (WHI) Study found that the use of Prempro, one of the popular synthetic hormone replacement medications at the time, increased the risk for breast cancer, heart disease, stroke, and blood clots. It looked as though the cure was worse than the problem it had been meant to correct! Millions of women panicked and immediately tossed out their HRT prescriptions. That may have been a bit hasty. Here are the key concepts to understand in regard to the WHI study:

- There was no individualized testing of the hormone needs of participants. They took a one-size-fits-all approach. In psychiatry, this is like giving all depressed patients Prozac, which works about as well as giving everyone sugar pills.
- The synthetic hormones that were tested were not cycled like your body's natural hormones.
- Estrone (associated with a higher incidence of breast cancer) was in high concentration in HRT formulations.
- Equilenin, or horse mare estrogen, also in the formula, is not easy for your body to recognize, and its metabolites can create significant damage to DNA.
- Taking oral estrogens has been found to increase C-reactive protein, an inflammatory marker that is associated with increased cancer and heart disease risk. This same risk does not seem to apply to bioidentical transdermal (topical) estradiol.
- Progestins (synthetic progesterone) have a long list of side effects associated with them. Progestins do not function in the body the same way as bioidentical progesterone. For example, progestins increase breast cancer risk whereas bioidentical progesterone will lower breast cancer risk.

So when you look at the problems highlighted in the WHI study, they were specific for the type of hormones given (synthetic) and how they were given. But the result was that the study led to all hormone replacement being condemned. The media incited a fear in women that has potentially done more harm than good.

Another problem seen with the use of synthetic female sex hormones is drug-induced nutrient depletion. Synthetic estrogen replacement therapy can deplete the key nutrients, such as vitamin B_6 and magnesium. Magnesium helps balance glucose and insulin regulation. Vitamin B_6 is involved in the production of serotonin for mood and appetite control. The synthetic progestins can cause the depletion of many nutrients including B vitamins, tyrosine, CoQ10, vitamin E, and folic acid. Taking synthetic HRT by mouth can also increase imbalances in the natural gut flora, causing increases in *Candida* (yeast) populations. This can lead not only to vaginal yeast disturbances, but it can put significant stress on your immune system too.

I have seen estrogen, progesterone, and testosterone replacement with bioidentical hormones have tremendous value when done correctly. BHRT is the use of sex hormones derived from either plant sources (usually soy and wild yam) or processed from plant-based compounds by compounding pharmacists. Bioidentical hormones are exactly the same (molecularly) as those found in your body, and as such they are accepted and metabolized as if your body made them—producing the same physiologic responses as those of the body's natural hormones. When used properly, BHRT can bring hormones back to a normal level and alleviates uncomfortable symptoms of deficiency. Bioidentical estrogens will often be prescribed for women after blood, saliva, and urine testing show deficiencies. BHRT has been found to be effective in reducing the number and intensity of hot flashes and in improving sleep and other negative symptoms of perimenopause and menopause.

But are there risks? The primary risk to be concerned about in hormonal replacement for women is breast cancer. Low progesterone-to-estrogen ratios play an important role in that risk. If a woman has low progesterone levels, it is correlated with a fivefold increased risk of premenopausal breast cancer. And progesterone cream has been found to reduce the overproliferation of cells in breast tissue. This protective, antiproliferative effect of bioidentical progesterone is not seen with synthetic progestins.

Compared to the increased risks for cognitive decline while on HRT, natural progesterone has been found to enhance the repair processes in the brain, help with reducing anxiety, improve sleep patterns, and preserve cognitive function with age.

So far, the studies on BHRT are limited, but they do look promising. One French study looked at over three thousand women using natural progesterone and estradiol. This study found no increased health risks. Another larger French study compared women using HRT to women using BHRT and found that those using HRT had significantly greater risk of developing breast cancer than those on BHRT.

When used properly, here are some of the benefits I have seen of BHRT for women:

- Reduced or eliminated hot flashes
- Decreased vaginal dryness
- Improved skin elasticity
- Improved energy and blood flow
- Accelerated fat burning for improved weight loss
- Reduced sleep disturbances (insomnia and night sweats)
- Reduced emotional disturbances (mood swings, depression, nervousness, irritability, anxiousness)
- Reduced breast problems reduced (tenderness, fibrocystosis, etc.)
- Improved libido and sex drive
- Improved mental acuity (lapses of memory, foggy thinking, concentration, etc.)
- Reduced incontinence

Without knowing your true hormonal status through appropriate testing, it's impossible to get to the best balance for you. The reason BHRT may not work in some individuals is due to their health habits or the result of all their hormones not being balanced. For example, just balancing the sex hormones will not work if you are under chronic stress and your body is making excess cortisol. The excess cortisol can disrupt your metabolism, leading to further imbalances in sex hormones and other hormones like thyroid.

Natural Supplements to Alleviate Symptoms

The North American Menopause Society specifically recommends dietary isoflavones (found in soy and linseed products), black cohosh, and vitamin E for menopausal symptoms. Of all the available supplements, black cohosh is the only one to be consistently found to offer relief from hot flashes. While its long-term safety has not been determined, it seems fine for short-term use. Also, phytoestrogens, found in many foods, seem to offer help. Good sources are nuts and oilseeds (like flaxseed oil). There is also interesting new work that shows that DHEA, discussed in the next part, can significantly improve sexual function in menopausal women.

PART TWO: BALANCE THYROID, CORTISOL, DHEA, AND INSULIN

Low thyroid doesn't kill you. It just makes you wish you were dead."

—RICHARD AND KARILEE SHAMES, *THYROID MIND POWER*

THYROID

Anne is a once-in-a-lifetime teacher. She is firm, kind, creative, smart, and organized, and she has consistently earned the love and admiration of her students and parents year after year. Having been a child and adult psychiatrist for decades, I have seen many excellent teachers and many not-so-excellent ones. Anne is at the top of my list. She was my daughter's second-grade teacher.

When Anne confided to my wife, Tana, that she wanted to see me because she was feeling tired, in a mental fog, and felt like she had ADD, even though she never had symptoms of it in the past, I was willing to help. She was a vegetarian but complained of being sensitive to many foods and said that whenever she drank alcohol it would double her over in pain. If something in the morning set her off, she felt "out of skew" and irritable for the rest of the day. In addition, she was sensitive to loud sounds and felt anxious a lot of the time. Her anxiety and the tendency to replay things over and over again in her mind kept her from being able to relax. Sometimes she found that she worried for days at a time.

One of the first things I did was check her important numbers. It turned out that she had very high levels of thyroid antibodies: Her thyroid peroxidase antibodies were fewer than 1,000, when normal is fewer than 35. Having such a high level of thyroid antibodies meant that Anne had an autoimmune condition in which her body was attacking her own thyroid tissue. Anne also had a very low vitamin D level, which is essential to the health of many organs, including the thyroid.

Using our Amen Clinics Four Circles Approach, plus getting Anne's vitamin D level optimized and getting her thyroid properly treated, made a big difference in helping her focus and increasing her energy. She didn't have ADD or any other such condition. Like many women, Anne needed her hormones balanced in a holistic way.

WHEN A GOOD THYROID GOES BAD, THE BRAIN SUFFERS

Reproductive hormones aren't the only hormones that affect how you look and feel and think. Among the most influential are the hormones produced in your neck by your thyroid gland.

Too little thyroid, and you feel like a slug. Hypothyroidism makes you feel like you just want to lie on the couch all day with a bag of chips.

Everything works slower, including your heart, your bowels, and your brain. When we perform SPECT scans of people with hypothyroidism, we see decreased brain activity. Many other studies confirm that overall low brain function in hypothyroidism leads to depression, cognitive impairment, anxiety, and feelings of being in a mental fog. The thyroid gland drives the production of many neurotransmitters that run the brain, such as serotonin, dopamine, adrenaline, and noradrenaline. A low thyroid can cause a compensatory rise in the adrenal hormones of adrenaline, which makes you feel wired, and cortisol, the hormone of stress. So people feel tired, wired, and stressed at the same time. In one group of patients with rapid cycling bipolar disorder, more than 50 percent had hypothyroidism. Experts conservatively estimate that one-third of all depressions are directly related to thyroid imbalance. More than 80 percent of people with low-grade hypothyroidism have impaired memory function.

Low thyroid is associated with a host of symptoms and problems, such as:

- Feeling cold when others are hot
- Weight gain
- Constipation
- Fatigue
- High cholesterol
- High blood pressure
- Dry, thinning, or losing hair, especially the eyebrows, where the outer third are often missing
- Dry skin
- Dry eyes
- Thin, cracking, or peeling nails
- Menstrual irregularities
- Endometriosis
- Infertility

- Recurrent miscarriages
- Birth defects
- Terrible menopause

Even if your thyroid is producing low-normal thyroid levels, you can still have symptoms known as subclinical hypothyroidism. If you're tired all the time, have gained weight, have dry skin, feel spacey, suffer from depression, feel cold all the time, and have a body temperature that tends to be lower than 98.6, you could have an underactive thyroid.

An overactive thyroid, or hyperthyroidism, is also a problem, because now everything in your body works too fast, including your heart, your bowels, and your digestion. It's like you're in hyperdrive. You feel jittery and edgy, as though you've had too much caffeine. If you suffer from sleeplessness, anxiety, irritability, racing thoughts, a fast pulse, breathlessness, weight loss despite an increased appetite, feeling too hot for no clear reason, and always feeling as though somebody set the thermostat too high, you could have an overactive thyroid. In extreme cases, you might see the classic systems of a goiter (a growth on the thyroid), weight loss, bulging eyes, and an intense staring gaze.

Your thyroid is a small butterfly-shaped gland located in your lower neck. When your doctor runs her hands along the base of your throat, she's checking to see if there are any noticeable problems with the size of your thyroid. But you can't really tell what's going on without a blood test. And it can take some adjusting to get your thyroid optimized. The main thyroid hormones—TSH, T3, and T4— all have to be in the right balance. It is estimated that tens of millions of people worldwide (5–25 percent of the world's population) have thyroid problems. Thyroid problems are more common as we age and they seem to be increasing in the population. In their book, *Thyroid Mind Power,* Richard and Karilee Shames report that "the last 40 years have witnessed a massive increase in the amount of hormone-disrupting synthetic chemicals, finding their way into our air, food and water. . . . The most sensitive and highly susceptible of human tissues turned out to be the thyroid gland."

Most thyroid issues are autoimmune, which means that the body is attacking itself. This can be due to the environmental toxins that are stored in our bodies or allergies to the food we eat (gluten and milk products in particular) or to something in the air we breathe. Many physicians consider the thyroid to be the "canary in the coal mine." That is, the suspicion is that the recent skyrocketing rates of hypothyroidism may be related to ingested toxins interfering with the peripheral conversion of T4 to T3.

Thyroid problems can occur at any time in a woman's life. But having a baby is an especially vulnerable time. During pregnancy, certain parts of the immune system relax so that immune cells and antibodies will not reject the baby's placenta, which is attached to the mother's uterus. This is why many women with thyroid problems feel that pregnancy is the best time of their lives. Being pregnant calms their thyroid issues. This happened to my wife, who has suffered with thyroid cancer and Hashimoto's disease, an autoimmune disease that affects the thyroid. Like many women with thyroid issues, she said that she felt better being pregnant than at any other time in her life.

After nine months, the situation changes. The baby is delivered, the placenta detaches, and parts of the immune system that were turned down to prevent early rejection of the placenta are now turned back up with a surge. It is well documented that thyroid problems are very common within six months of giving birth. According to researchers from Prague's Charles University, 35 percent of women who produce thyroid antibodies go on to have abnormal thyroid levels two years after giving birth.

Having thyroid problems when you're struggling with a two-year-old child is a prescription for disaster. Studies show that approximately

70 percent of women who were hypothyroid in the postpartum period were more careless, making significantly more mistakes in the care of their babies than women whose thyroid function was normal.

Nearly half of the women with postpartum hypothyroidism had significant nightmares compared to only 5 percent of women with normal thyroid function.

Thyroid problems are a major cause of postpartum depression, anxiety, and psychosis. In one study, 80–90 percent of postpartum depression was associated with thyroid abnormalities. And without effective thyroid treatment it is impossible to get well.

Postpregnancy is not the only vulnerable time for thyroid issues. It has been estimated that one in every four postmenopausal women has thyroid imbalances. According to the Ridha Arem, M.D., editor of the journal *Thyroid*, nearly 45 percent of people over age fifty have some degree of thyroid gland inflammation. Dr. Arem suggests that minor thyroid problems cause more disability in the elderly population than in the young, who have greater reserve. As we age, the thyroid, like many other active organs, becomes vulnerable to trouble.

Checking your thyroid can be done with a blood test. Don't settle for just a TSH test, which only measures your thyroid-stimulating hormone. These levels can be normal even while you have an undiagnosed thyroid problem. Instead, if you have any symptoms, insist your doctor order the following tests:

- TSH (according to the American Association of Clinical Endocrinologists, anything over 3.0 is abnormal and needs further investigation)
- Free T3 (active)
- Free T4 (inactive)

- Thyroid antibodies
  - Thyroid peroxidase antibodies
  - Thyroglobulin antibodies
- Liver function tests. Ninety-five percentof T4 is "activated" in the liver, so having a healthy liver is essential.
- Ferritin level. Ferritin is like the bus that drives the active T3 into the cells for the activity to occur. Ferritin needs to be above 90 for this to occur.

If your doctor refuses to order these tests, see someone else, or order them yourself at websites such as SaveOnLabs.com. Consider Bernadette's story:

Hi Dr. Amen:

I am a healthy, active thirty-two-year-old female who is very adamant on getting my yearly health and dental checkups, screenings and blood work. I have recently listened to (and read) Change Your Brain, Change Your Body, *and I believe wholeheartedly in your methods and helpful tips and tricks to stay well.*

I recently took your suggestion and had the more in-depth preliminary blood tests done (thyroid, hormones, vitamins, etc.), even though I was questioned by my doctor about why I wanted these ancillary tests when there was no apparent reason for conducting such research. I stated that I wanted to understand my numbers more than just what is happening in my vascular system.

Upon receiving the results of my blood work, I found that my "thyroglobulin antibodies" were high, indicating there was a problem. I immediately saw an endocrinologist, who did an ultrasound and found a 1.6 cm growth on my thyroid. The biopsy revealed I have papillary thyroid cancer, which has spread to my lymph nodes. If it hadn't been for your advice, this issue may have gone undiagnosed for some time and worsened my prognosis. Without reading your book, I may not have had a chance to write this email.

Thank you so much for what you do!

Sincerely,
Bernadette (get your important numbers checked!)

Factors That Inhibit Thyroid
- Excess stress and cortisol production
- Selenium deficiency
- Deficient protein, excess sugar
- Chronic illness
- Compromised liver or kidney function
- Cadmium, mercury, lead toxicity
- Herbicides, pesticides
- Oral contraceptives, excessive estrogen production

If you have thyroid issues, they can be effectively treated with a number of thyroid medications. Your doctor needs to test your levels regularly to make sure you are not taking too much or too little. There are also a number of natural dietary supplements that support thyroid function, including the herb rosemary, zinc, chromium, potassium, iodine, L-tyrosine, vitamins A, B_2, B_3, B_6, C, D, selenium, seaweed, and ashwagandha. Also, make sure to have healthy testosterone, insulin, and melatonin levels.

Let me state clearly that while these thyroid tests can be helpful, in the final analysis *your doctor, not the blood test, should diagnose you.* I have seen too many hypothyroid patients not treated by their physicians because their thyroid numbers were low but "within normal limits." It's a little like saying a vitamin D level of 31 is normal (normal range is 30–100). I have never wanted to be at the bottom of any class I was in. How a patient feels and functions (e.g., energy, constipation, dry hair, dry skin, cognition, body temperature) is more important in assessing thyroid function than just using arbitrary blood test normal ranges.

CORTISOL AND DHEA: OUR LADY OF PERPETUAL STRESS

We hear a lot of talk these days about adrenal fatigue, especially among women who are busy, stressed, and anxious. Is it possible for an organ to just wear itself out? Yes, it is. The adrenals are a pair of triangle-shaped glands that sit on top of your kidneys, and they are critically involved in your body's reaction to stress. The adrenals produce the hormones adrenaline, DHEA, and cortisol. Perhaps you've heard of the fight-or-flight response. It's the adrenals that put you in one of these lifesaving modes by releasing these chemicals.

For example, suppose you're hiking through the woods with your children when you see a mountain lion; immediately your adrenals start producing adrenaline and the other hormones you need to give you the burst of energy you can use to either fight the lion or pick up the children and run away as fast as you can. The problem is, your body doesn't really recognize the difference between one kind of stress and another. Whether it's physical stress at the sight of the lion or mental stress caused by your raging teenager or catty co-workers, your body reacts the same way, pumping out those chemicals.

When you run away from the lion, you process the chemicals and get them out of your system. But when you get stressed over the way your co-worker looked at you, all you can do is go back to your office and stew. That leaves a dangerous cocktail of chemicals surging through your body until they're finally metabolized.

In today's world, you're probably faced with that kind of psychological stress on a daily basis. You wake up to a blaring alarm, and the first thing you do is check your email to see what people are demanding of you now. Then it's rushing off to work, getting stopped in bumper-to-bumper traffic, and arriving late to face a slew of impossible deadlines. Then the school calls to tell you that your son has been getting into fights. On and on it goes, causing your poor adrenals to keep pumping out cortisol and other chemicals that your body doesn't know what to do with.

Cortisol is made from progesterone. So if you make lots of cortisol, progesterone levels go down along with estrogen. Women could forever try to balance out estrogen and progesterone, but without managing cortisol, they can never get to a stable pattern of sex hormone. With elevations in cortisol, blood sugar and insulin levels also rise. And, your brain doesn't fare well. Serotonin (the "calming" brain chemical) levels drop leading to anxiety, nervousness, or depression. Food cravings will also increase and your health can spiral out of control. Chronic exposure to stress hormones has been shown to kill cells in your hippocampus, one of the major memory centers in the brain, especially when DHEA is also low.

This goes on for months and years, and finally the adrenal glands can just get tired. When they do, we call it adrenal fatigue, and now your body doesn't have the resources it needs to deal with all that daily stress. You can barely get out of bed in the morning or get yourself through the day.

You could also be getting fat. Adrenal fatigue leads to an especially dangerous buildup of fat in your abdomen. Not only do you ruin your chances for a flat belly, but you're at greater risk for cardiovascular disease and diabetes too. Low cortisol also promotes inflammation, alters blood sugar control, affects immune function, and alters sex hormone production. When the adrenals are busy making stress hormones, it depletes the reservoir of DHEA, which should have eventually been converted to sex hormones.

Doctors are seeing patients with adrenal fatigue more frequently lately, and a big reason is that so many of us are skimping on sleep. The human body needs sleep, about seven to eight hours every night, and if it doesn't get it, your system automatically goes into a stress state. Then, you self-medicate to counteract the lack of sleep, and just make things worse. Drinking coffee or caffeinated energy drinks to keep yourself awake adds to the stress load. Taking some alcohol in the evening to quiet down after all that caffeine may be a temporary fix. But once the alcohol wears off, it puts your body into another stress response that wakes you up at two in the morning. Then you can't sleep and you need more caffeine to meet the next day. Now you're in a never-ending cycle of stress that exhausts your adrenal system and keeps you operating on the edge, and never at your best.

How do you know if you might be suffering from adrenal fatigue? Here are some common symptoms:

- Decreased ability to withstand stress
- Morning and afternoon fatigue, lack of stamina
- High blood pressure and rapid heartbeat
- Abdominal fat that doesn't go away no matter what you do
- Mental fog with poor memory and difficulty concentrating
- Low libido
- Craving for sweets or salty foods
- Hypoglycemic under stress
- Dizziness when getting up from a sitting or lying position
- Signs of premature aging
- Lowered resistance to infection
- Poor wound healing.

From Dr. Tami Meraglia, an integrative medicine physician in Seattle, who sees many stressed-out women:

My patients have an "aha" moment when I explain the difference between stress, lack of stress, and doing things that repair the damage and inflammation created by stress. Most patients think that going home and "relaxing" is healing the stress from the day. It is not. That is merely the lack of stress, if you are lucky. My patients

*see results when they actively engage in activities like the meditation
exercises on your online site to heal and rejuvenate the damage done
by the stress of that day. I remember asking my dentist when I was
eleven years old if I had to floss all my teeth. He told me only the
ones I wanted to keep. I think meditation is similar. Stress damages
our health every day. You only need to meditate on the days that you
want to heal that damage.*

To properly test for adrenal fatigue, you or your doctor can check
your levels of cortisol with a saliva test and DHEA-S with a blood test.
Saliva cortisol levels should be measured four times during the day:
when you first wake up, around lunchtime, around dinnertime, and
just before you go to sleep. Ideally, your cortisol levels are high in the
morning, to wake you up, and taper off slowly during the day and evening, allowing you to fall into a restful sleep at night. When cortisol
levels are too high, you feel wired. When they are too low, you feel exhausted, spacey, or sluggish.

> *It's possible to have cortisol levels that are too high for some por-
> tions of the day and too low for others. So a four-point test is
> needed to see what the situation is.*

DHEA is a natural precursor hormone secreted by the adrenal
glands, ovaries, and the brain. It produces estrogen and, to a lesser extent, testosterone. DHEA also protects brain cells from the beta-amyloid
protein that is associated with Alzheimer's. Studies show that higher
levels of DHEA as you age are associated with longevity. Peak levels
are typically reached when men and women are in their thirties; they
then begin to lose approximately 2 percent per year. During periods of
chronic stress, the release of the stress hormone cortisol can decrease
levels of DHEA, lowering immunity and potentially accelerating the
aging processes.

Studies have found that DHEA therapy in women with adrenal fatigue can also help boost a low libido during menopause. Low levels of DHEA have also been linked to weight gain and depression.

One of the most important reasons to measure DHEA is that low levels in combination with high cortisol levels put you at risk for memory loss. Originally it was thought that high cortisol was the culprit in damaging the hippocampus, the brain's major learning and memory center, but new studies report that people with Alzheimer's have lower DHEA levels. When DHEA drops, the protective effects of DHEA on the brain are lost.

If your DHEA is low, it can be easily supplemented. There is good evidence that validates DHEA supplementation to help support adrenal gland function, mood, and your weight. Generally, we start with 10 mg and go up from there. DHEA is usually well tolerated, but there can be some unpleasant side effects like acne and facial hair owing to the tendency of DHEA to increase testosterone levels. These can be avoided by using a specific metabolite of DHEA called 7-Keto-DHEA. It is more expensive than simple DHEA, but it may be preferable in some cases. The dose of 7-Keto-DHEA is typically between 50 and 100 mg.

A more serious concern with DHEA is that it partly converts itself into sex hormones like testosterone and estrogen. While this is actually a good thing for healthy individuals who want to stave off aging, it can be a problem to women who have had hormone-dependent cancers, such as breast or ovarian cancers. In these cases, 7-Keto-DHEA can be a better solution. If you think DHEA supplementation could be helpful to you, make sure to talk to a health care professional who is experienced using hormone therapies.

Natural supplements can also help. For example, B vitamins support the adrenal system and can help you deal with stress. 5-HTP is a calming supplement that boosts serotonin levels and can support sleep, so that you feel less stress, which can also help with weight loss. Also, L-theanine (200 mg two or three times a day), Relora (750mg two to three times a day), magnesium, holy basil (200–400 mg two to three times a day), ashwagandha (250 mg two to three times a day), and rhodiola (200 mg two to three times a day) have been shown to be useful.

Adrenal fatigue can also be helped by natural stress-management techniques, such as laughter, deep breathing exercises, and regular relaxation exercises. Learning how to meditate, recognize and correct negative thinking patterns (more on this in chapter 6), or use self-hypnosis can calm jittery nerves.

Insulin

Having healthy insulin levels is one of the major keys to a clear mind and a healthy female body. Insulin is a hormone that unlocks cell membranes so that they can absorb glucose and other nutrients. When insulin levels are high, the body stores fat instead of breaking it down. Insulin is secreted by the pancreas in response to carbohydrates. Simple sugars and highly processed carbohydrates, such as baked goods, candy, bread, pasta, and crackers, demand a large release of insulin from the pancreas and can cause significant blood sugar highs and lows.

Low blood sugar levels can make you feel foggy and sluggish. High blood sugar levels, over time, are a disaster for your brain and body, causing blood vessels to become brittle and easily broken. Insulin dysregulation can lead to diabetes, which harms every organ in the body and can lead to depression, dementia, and a wide variety of illnesses. I have seen family members and friends with diabetes lose limbs and eyesight, and develop heart disease and dementia. Like the others, you want to have great respect for and optimize this hormone.

Test your blood sugar and insulin levels, and if they are abnormal, think of it as a health crisis to take very seriously. Eliminating sugar and other simple carbohydrates can help to regulate the body's production of insulin and allow fat to be broken down for energy. In addition, high consumption of sugar depletes chromium, a mineral that is needed by insulin receptors. Without chromium, insulin receptors cannot recognize insulin. Sugar does not add any nutritional benefit to your diet but instead depletes chromium and other valuable vitamins and minerals.

Type 1 diabetes occurs when the body refuses to make insulin; type 2 occurs when the body mismanages it. Recently, scientists have reported new evidence linking abnormal insulin levels to Alzheimer's disease. The correlation is so strong that some have labeled Alzheimer's "type 3" diabetes. It was recently discovered that cells in the hippocampus actually produce insulin. The hippocampus is one of the first areas in the brain to die in Alzheimer's. Besides converting food into energy, the brain has other uses for insulin, including helping with learning and making new memories. Brain cells have special receptors for insulin, which it uses when making new memories. Insulin resistance in these cells can cause a downward cognitive cycle. A 2009 study showed that giving intranasal insulin to people with mild cognitive impairment or early Alzheimer's helped memory and attention and it helped to decrease the clumps of toxic chemicals thought to cause Alzheimer's.

Getting your insulin and blood sugar levels optimized will help not only your waistline, but also your ability to learn and remember your husband's name.

Fasting insulin and blood sugar levels, and HgA1c should be tested on a regular basis.

Diet Is Crucial in Insulin Regulation—To reverse insulin resistance, eliminate all simple sugars, wheat (including whole wheat), and processed foods and eat a diet high in smart carbohydrates, which are high in fiber and low on the GI. Without the constant intake of simple sugars and high glycemic carbohydrates, the pancreas is not called upon to constantly secrete high levels of insulin. Without these high levels of insulin, cells become more insulin-sensitive. Eating fiber-rich whole grains can slow the release of blood glucose and the rise of insulin, but until your blood sugar is under control, it is better to eliminate them. A Swedish study compared the effects on blood sugar of a grain-free diet (the Paleo diet) compared to the Mediterranean diet, a diet that allows only whole grains, among other healthy foods. After twelve weeks, the blood sugar rise was markedly lower in the Paleolithic group (–26%), whereas it barely changed in the Mediterranean group (–7%). At the end of the study, all patients in the Paleolithic group had normal blood glucose.

Another reason whole grains may impact weight and insulin resistance is that they contain proteins called lectins, which some researchers suspect can promote inflammation and halt weight-loss efforts. Aside from promoting weight loss and improving blood sugar regulation, avoiding grains is very beneficial for overall intestinal health. Anti-inflammatory in nature, the Paleo diet promotes a favorable balance of good to bad bacteria in the gut. Many patients feel relief from minor digestive discomforts such as bloating, gas, and indigestion when following a low sugar, no-dairy, no-grain plan.

Insulin resistance is closely related to metabolic syndrome, a cluster of conditions—hypertension, high blood sugar levels, high cholesterol, and belly fat—that together increase your risk of heart disease, stroke, and diabetes. Adhering to a diet that includes only smart carbohydrates, healthy fats and proteins, and eliminates grains, potatoes, rice, sugar, and processed food is essential to reversing disease. Losing as little as 10 percent of your belly fat can decrease cardiovascular risk by 75 percent.

Managing Your Blood Sugar Is Critical to Looking and Feeling Young—Studies have found that insulin resistance is a predictor of many age-related diseases. Once insulin is elevated, it can reduce the production of DHEA, which is needed to build sex hormones. And when insulin stimulates belly fat production, the *fat accumulation can alter hormone function, by turning tes-*

tosterone into toxic estrogens. Insulin resistance is also associated with inflammation.

There is another way that insulin resistance can accelerate the aging process. It can lead to glycation— a process in which glucose reacts with protein in an undesired way. This reaction results in sugar-damaged proteins (similar to browning food in the oven) appropriately called advanced glycation end products (AGEs). The formation of AGEs happens in everyone and is a major factor in the aging process itself. However, AGE formation is increased under the conditions of hormonal imbalances, oxidative stress, and insulin resistance. AGEs may lead to premature signs of aging like wrinkles and brown spots and may eventually lead to the development of type 2 diabetes, cataracts, macular degeneration, kidney disease, cardiovascular diseases, and even cancer.

Insulin resistance can be improved with dietary changes and the use of dietary supplements like magnesium, bitter melon extract, and chromium. The mineral magnesium plays a critical role in carbohydrate metabolism and preventing metabolic syndrome. Magnesium seems to influence the release and activity of insulin and help balance glucose levels. Testosterone replacement has a significant impact on improving blood sugar and reversing the trend toward insulin resistance.

BALANCING YOUR HORMONES NATURALLY

As I've suggested throughout this chapter, there are many well-established, natural steps you can take to balance your hormones. Here are three simple ones.

1. Hormone Envy—As I mentioned in chapter 1, having brain envy is the first critical step to unleashing the power of the female brain. You have to care about the health of your brain. Likewise, to have a great brain, you have to care about the health of your hormones. Make optimizing them a priority and your life will be so much happier.

2. Avoid Bad—To keep all of your hormones healthy, it is critical to avoid anything that hurts or diminishes them, such as synthetic chemicals, stress, processed food, high sugar, a bad-fat diet, wheat, a lack of sleep, cigarettes, excessive caffeine, more than a few glasses of alcohol a week, low vitamin D levels, obesity, inflammation, poor muscle tone, and a lack of exercise.

Avoid toxins and toxic environments. Many of the chemicals and toxins we're exposed to every day can have a disturbing effect on our health. For example, research shows that perfluorochemicals, the chemicals found in nonstick cookware and some food packaging, are associated with endocrine disruption in women, leading to early menopause. The related chemicals perfluorooctanoic acid and perfluorooctane sulfonic acid are also found in cookware, stain guards, carpets, furniture, and paints. And chemicals like lead in your water can also be affecting you. Plus, have you read the list of ingredients on those body lotions you're using? Or the cleaners you're using all over the house? Many natural products are available for you to use instead. Try to avoid toxic chemicals as best you can, and protect your daughters from them, as they have been associated with early menstruation.

Don't smoke. Of course the biggest environmental pollutant you should avoid is cigarette smoke. Recent research confirms that smoking lowers the age of menopause. It's also associated with more severe hot flashes, specifically for its effects on sex hormone metabolism. Add to that the cardiovascular effects and relationship to lung cancer and it's impossible to ignore the truth: Smoking makes you sick.

Be careful with your weight. A study of Spanish women confirms the fact that being obese adds to the severity of menopausal symptoms. Obesity is also related to diseases, such as diabetes. We've all heard (and perhaps seen firsthand) that weight gain creeps up on us as we get older. Studies show that obesity, especially with visceral fat distribution, and mortality are directly related in middle-aged women. It may be that as women age and experience progressive declines in many hormones, such as the estrogens and DHEA, this leads to altered body composition and the associated weight gain. This, in turn, leads to metabolic disturbances and increased incidence of mortality.

I know it's hard to watch everything you eat when you're feeling tired and depressed. In chapter 5, I will give you a very specific plan on how to feed your female brain to optimize your health. Eat a brain-smart diet and you will look and feel younger and see results in as little as two weeks.

Reduce inflammation. You may be suffering from chronic inflammation and not even realize it. Persistent exposure to free radicals from processed vegetable oils in fried food, powdered coffee creamer, cookies, crackers, and all those other processed foods we eat are one aggravating cause. Then there's the exposure to heavy metals, pesticides, and other toxins in our environment. Or you could have a low-grade infection, the result of an old injury, root canal, or failure to get your teeth cleaned. Depending on your unique genetic makeup, the resulting chronic inflammation can lead to vascular disease, Alzheimer's, diabetes, arthritis, bowel problems, and cancer.

If you have chronic inflammation, now is the time to do everything you can to eliminate this dangerous condition. Clean up your diet and your environment. Take omega-3s and other anti-inflammatory oils, like olive oil. Stay away from processed foods, additives, and artificial ingredients. Reduce your intake of alcohol and caffeine. Don't smoke. And find out if you have allergies to dairy, gluten, soy, nuts, and other reactive foods. Also, exercise and get plenty of sleep. Don't use the excuse that you don't have the time. That's an excuse that could be killing you.

3. Do Good—Help keep your hormones in balance with physical exercise, including weight training, appropriate sleep, a healthy diet, as described in chapter 5, and a clean environment.
Exercise. Physical activity is important for helping you get through

difficult times for a number of reasons. First, it raises levels of serotonin, the neurotransmitter that makes you feel good. Second, it improves your circulation. More blood to your brain makes you less foggy, and more blood to your sex organs keeps them functioning at their best. Third, it helps you control your weight by burning calories and suppressing your appetite, provided you don't "reward" yourself after exercising with a cinnamon bun and double latte. Women have to be careful about that because they have been shown to increase their calorie intake after exercise, which undoes all the good of it. By the way, there's been fascinating research that indicates that yoga is an especially effective exercise at reducing menopausal symptoms like hot flashes and night sweats. If you are in the earlier stages of adrenal distress, exercise can help you burn off the anxiety and extra cortisol. But if you are in the "fatigued" stage, take it easy. Women whose cortisol levels are too low shouldn't be pushing themselves too hard. In fact, I never recommend my patients push themselves too hard. Consistent, reasonable exercise is the key.

The regimen I give my patients is very simple. Walk like you're late for forty-five minutes four times a week. The faster you walk as you age, the less likely you are to die earlier. Also, lift light weights. The stronger you are as you age, the less likely you are to get Alzheimer's disease. In addition, weight lifting has been shown to boost testosterone levels. But do not hurt yourself or let anyone else hurt you. If you are with a trainer who is yelling at you to lift heavier and heavier weights, fire him or her and get someone who is reasonable.

Get enough sleep. You know that when you don't get enough sleep you feel groggy, listless, and irritable. And that's just what you see on the surface. Lack of sleep affects your brain chemistry and has been shown to interfere with hippocampal-dependent memory, something you don't need when you're already suffering from brain fog. Also, interesting new research indicates that REM (rapid eye movement sleep—the kind you have when you're dreaming) is especially important for the health of the neural cytoskeleton, the structure supporting your neurons. And lack of sleep has long been associated with weight gain. A minimum of seven nightly hours of sleep seems to be the most effective amount.

Eat a healthy diet. Eating a healthy diet is important at every stage of your life. But during menopause, in particular, you want your food to help you feel better, not put your body under additional strain. Stay away from processed foods as much as possible and eat balanced meals, following the plan I share with you in chapter 5.

Keep your environment clean. Toxic chemicals are all around us, for example in the toiletries we use on our own bodies and the cleaning solutions we apply around our homes. Read labels and try to find less toxic alternatives wherever you can.

KEY VITAMINS, MINERALS, AND HERBS FOR HORMONE BALANCE

To Support Multiple or All Hormones

- Multiple vitamin
- Fish oil (2,000 mg a day)
- Probiotics for gut health to bind bad estrogens (10 billion–60 billion colony-supporting units [CFUs])
- Calcium citrate (400–500 mg twice a day) and chelated magnesium (200–300 mg twice a day), to keep your nerves calm
- Vitamin D (2,000 international units (IU) of vitamin D daily generally, but it's important to get tested individually) to get the most benefit from calcium
- Zinc for testosterone and thyroid 15 mg
- Melatonin (1–6 mg)
- Selenium (200 µg)

To Balance Estrogen

- DIM (100–200 mg a day)
- Calcium d-glucarate (500 mg a day)

- Plant phytoestrogens, including black cohosh (20–80 mg twice daily)
- Flaxseeds
- Evening primrose oil (500 mg twice a day)
- Black cohosh (20–80 mg twice a day)

To alleviate PMS

- Calcium citrate (400–500 mg twice a day)
- Chelated magnesium (200–300 mg twice a day)
- Vitamin A, B complex with 50 mg of B_6
- Evening primrose oil (500 mg twice a day)
- 5-HTP (50–100 mg twice a day) to possibly boost serotonin and decrease anxiety and worry
- Green tea (600 mg twice a day) or L-tyrosine (500 mg two to three times a day) for focus
- Vitex/chasteberry (20–40 mg a day to improve PMS symptoms; has a progesterone-like effect

To Balance Testosterone

- DHEA (depending on lab test needs)
- Zinc (15 mg)
- Saw palmetto to drive down high levels of testosterone

To Balance Thyroid

- Zinc (15 mg)
- L-tyrosine (500 mg two to three times a day)
- Herb rosemary
- Chromium (100–400 µg/day)
- Potassium
- Iodine
- Vitamins A, B_2, B_3, B_6, C, D
- Seaweed
- Ashwagandha (250–500 mg once or twice a day)

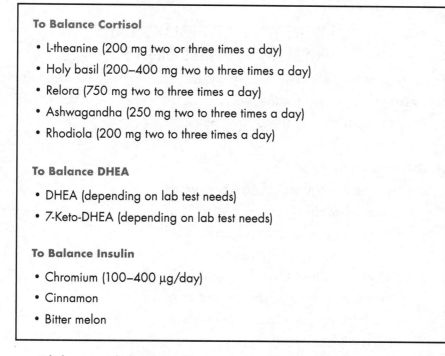

To Balance Cortisol

- L-theanine (200 mg two or three times a day)
- Holy basil (200–400 mg two to three times a day)
- Relora (750 mg two to three times a day)
- Ashwagandha (250 mg two to three times a day)
- Rhodiola (200 mg two to three times a day)

To Balance DHEA

- DHEA (depending on lab test needs)
- 7-Keto-DHEA (depending on lab test needs)

To Balance Insulin

- Chromium (100–400 µg/day)
- Cinnamon
- Bitter melon

It's been said that your hormones make you who you are. But you have something to say about it too! You can make the choices that improve your hormone balance so you feel healthy, calm, and mentally sharp. And now is the perfect time to start making the new choices so you can start living your optimal life right now.

Hour 4 Exercise—Take the Hormone Questionnaires and Inventory Your Healthy and Unhealthy Hormone Habits

1. TAKE THE HORMONE QUESTIONNAIRES

Understanding and optimizing your hormone status is essential to unleashing the power of the female brain. Take the Amen Clinics Brain Hormone Questionnaires for Women at www.amensolution.com/fe malehormonequestionnaires. If there are any signs of trouble, we'll give you suggestions on what to do next, including when to see a professional.

2. INVENTORY YOUR HEALTHY AND UNHEALTHY HORMONE HABITS

From the lists below, circle those statements that apply to you. Use the information in this book, and especially this chapter, to help you create a strategy to address your unhealthy habits.

Healthy Hormone Habits
- Getting seven to eight hours of sleep every night
- Eating a healthy diet
- Eating low-glycemic, brain-smart carbs
- Eating fiber, especially lignins found in green beans, peas, and so on, to help bind unhealthy estrogens
- Drinking water (half your weight in ounces is a good rule of thumb for people under 250 pounds)
- Effectively managing stress
- Fostering healthy gut flora
- Maintaining a healthy cholesterol level, not too high or too low
- Exercising regularly and incorporating weight training into your exercise regimen
- Adding targeted nutrients and supplements to your diet

Unhealthy Hormone Habits
- Consuming alcohol (even small amounts in women have been shown to increase breast cancer risk so less is better)
- Ignoring allergies to milk or gluten
- Smoking
- Ignoring inflammation (high homocysteine or C-reactive protein levels)
- Indulging poor muscle tone
- Not exercising

- Consuming excessive caffeine (more than a cup or two a day increases stress hormones)
- Consuming excessive sugar
- Eating high glycemic carbs, including wheat
- Eating processed foods
- Eating diets low in fiber
- Consuming animal protein, grain-fed or raised with hormones or antibiotics
- Being overweight, especially belly fat (turns testosterone into estrogen)
- Experiencing chronic stress
- Experiencing adrenal fatigue
- Taking certain medications, such as birth control pills, antacid cimetidine
- Allowing unhealthy gut flora to flourish
- Allowing excessive yeast to flourish
- Eating from plastic containers
- Microwaving in plastic containers
- Using nonstick cookware that contains perfluorochemicals
- Using personal care items such as face creams, shampoos, and toiletries that contain estrogens and especially phthalates
- Allowing zinc deficiency
- Allowing selenium deficiency
- Exposing yourself to cadmium, mercury, lead toxicity
- Exposing yourself to herbicides and pesticides
- Fostering estrone production through consumption of excess sugar, the antacid cimetidine, birth control pills, hypothyroidism, smoking, and pesticide exposure

5

FEED THE FEMALE BRAIN:

FLATTEN YOUR TUMMY AND BOOST BRAIN
RESERVES BY HEALING YOUR GUT AND
EATING BRAIN-HEALTHY SUPERFOODS

*Getting your food right is the fifth step to unleashing
the power of the female brain.
Eating right is about abundance, not deprivation.
If we're not willing to settle for junk living, we certainly
shouldn't settle for junk food.*

—SALLY EDWARDS

Your brain uses 20–30 percent of the calories you consume. It is the most expensive real estate in your body. If you want your female brain and body to live longer, look younger, be smarter, and feel happier one of the most important things to do is get your nutrition right. There is simply no way around it. You can exercise all you want, think all the right thoughts, meditate, and take dietary supplements, but if you continue to eat highly processed foods laden with sugar, bad fats, and salt; made from ingredients grown with pesticides; flavored with artificial sweeteners; colored with artificial dyes; and preserved with artificial preservatives, there is just no way to keep your brain and body working at their peak. If your food is not the best, you will never be your best. This chapter is about helping you eat right to think right.

In my experience, when you get your diet right, it has the potential to carry over to help other people in your family, community, place of worship, and workplace. I have seen this happen repeatedly in my own practice and in my work with corporations and churches.

The typical Western diet, consisting on average of only fifteen different foods that contain an overabundance of bad fat, salt, and sugar—think cheeseburgers, fries, sodas, and candy bars—promotes inflammation and has been associated with depression, ADD, dementia, heart disease, cancer, diabetes, and obesity. Think of what a cheeseburger consists of: a beef patty, lettuce, tomato, cheese, pickles, onions on a sesame seed bun (that's two foods if you count the seeds separately from the bun), plus mustard, mayonnaise, and ketchup, plus a serving of French fries and giant-size cola, and you've got twelve foods right there and, for many, a full day's supply of fat, salt, *and* calories.

If you start making better food choices today, you will quickly notice that you have more energy, better focus, a better memory, better moods, and a flatter tummy. A number of new studies have reported that a healthy diet is associated with significantly lower risks of Alzheimer's disease and depression. Plus, what really surprises most women is that when they decide to get healthy, their food options get better, not worse. It is the start of a wonderful new relationship with food.

When it comes to food, so many people are like how I used to be—a yo-yo. Crave bad food . . . overeat it . . . feel lousy . . . then hate yourself after the fact. It is way too much drama. When you decide to get healthy and get control of your food, you will eat better than ever and it will affect everything in your life in a positive way.

Tana has written several amazing cookbooks to help support our patients and readers in their efforts to get healthy, and of course I get to try everything first. I love her breakfast protein smoothies, which are loaded with vegetables; lentil soup; rack of lamb; and turkey bolognaise. I feel smarter when I eat fresh wild salmon, and I love her stuffed red bell peppers. I don't want fast- or poor-quality food anymore because it makes me feel tired and stupid. I want the right foods that help me be at my smartest all the time, and I want that for you too. And, contrary to what most people think, eating in a brain-healthy way is not more expensive; it is less expensive. Your medical bills will be lower and your productivity will go way up. And what price can you put on feeling amazing? Moreover, eating in a healthy way is a sign of self-love. If you truly care about yourself, how can you put poor-quality, health-damaging calories into your body that promote illness?

Your mind-set here is critical. Ultimately, eating right is not about deprivation; it is about abundance. You will realize that spoiling yourself, and giving in to bad food cravings, is indeed spoiling your health and is definitely not the sign of a rational mind.

In this chapter, I am going to show you the Four Circles Approach to feeding the female brain.

- Biology
  - Nine rules of brain-healthy eating
  - Fifty-two best brain-healthy superfoods
  - How to manipulate your mind with food
  - Foods to boost mood, focus, motivation, and memory
  - How to heal your gut to boost your brain
- Psychology
  - Ways to make your thoughts around food helpful, instead of hurtful

- How to break the hurtful psychological food patterns from the past
- Social Connections
  - The health of the people with whom you eat significantly influences your longevity
- Spiritual Health
  - Honoring your food
  - Respecting and replenishing food sources for generations to come

THE FOUR CIRCLES APPROACH TO FEEDING THE FEMALE BRAIN

BIOLOGY

The Amen Clinics Nine Rules of Brain-Healthy Eating

If you are going to eat right to think right, it is critical to make sure your food is loaded with proper nutrients that your body is able to properly digest. Here are the nine rules we have refined and teach our patients at the Amen Clinics.

Rule 1. Eat "High-Quality Calories" but Not Too Many of Them—Don't let anyone tell you that calories don't count. They absolutely do. But it is not as simple as calories in versus calories out. I want you to think about eating mostly high-quality calories. One cinnamon roll can cost you 720 calories, and a small quiche can be more than 1,000 calories and will drain your brain, whereas a 400-calorie salad made of spinach, salmon, blueberries, apples, walnuts, and red bell peppers will supercharge your energy and make you smarter.

I think of calories like money, and I hate wasting money. If you have a high metabolism, like having a lot of money, you don't have to worry much about calories. If you have a low metabolism, which happens to a lot of us as we grow older, you have to be very wise in how you spend your calories.

The research about calories is very clear. If you eat more calories than you need, you will be fatter, sicker, and less productive. In one study, researchers followed a large group of rhesus monkeys for twenty years. The monkeys in one group ate all the food they wanted; those in another group ate 30 percent less. The monkeys that ate anything they wanted were three times more likely to suffer from cancer, heart disease, and diabetes; in addition, researchers saw significant shrinkage in the important decision-making areas of their brains. Further, the calorie-restricted monkeys had smoother skin and healthier hair.

If weight is an issue for you, it is a smart idea to know how many calories a day you need to either maintain or lose weight. The average active fifty-year-old woman needs about 1,800 calories a day. You also need to know how many calories a day you actually put in your body, just like you need to know how much money you spend. Overeating is the exact same thing as overspending. When you overeat you bankrupt your brain and your body. If weight is a problem for you, keep a journal just like you keep a checkbook. Start the day with the number of calories you can spend and have a sense of where you are throughout the day. And don't spend them all in one place! This strategy makes a huge difference for my patients. When they actually write down everything they eat for a month, it causes them to stop lying to themselves about their calories and overcome their "calorie amnesia."

In our online community (www.amensolution.com), there is a food journal to help you get started. Plus, in one of my favorite articles titled "100 Ways to Leave Your Blubber," we'll show you how to cut your calories by 30 percent without feeling hungry.

View "100 Ways to Leave Your Blubber"

Rule 2. Drink Plenty of Water and Avoid Liquid Calories—
Your brain is 80 percent water. Anything that dehydrates it, such as too much caffeine or alcohol, decreases your thinking and impairs your judgment. Make sure you get plenty of water every day.

On a trip to New York City I saw a poster that read "Are You Pouring on the Pounds . . . Don't Drink Yourself Fat." I thought it was brilliant. A study found that on average Americans drink 450 calories a day, twice as many as we did thirty years ago. Just adding the extra 225 calories a day will put 23 pounds of fat a year on your body and most people tend *not* to count the calories they drink. Did you know that some coffee drinks or some cocktails, such as margaritas, can cost you more than 700 calories? One very simple strategy that can help you lose a lot of weight is to eliminate most of the calories you drink.

My favorite drink is water mixed with a little lemon juice and a little bit of the natural sweetener stevia. It tastes like lemonade, so I feel like I'm spoiling myself, and it has virtually no calories. And many of my patients make spa water and really feel like they are spoiling themselves. Spa water is water with a few cucumber slices, lemons, or strawberries in it.

Rule 3. Eat High-Quality Lean Protein Throughout the Day—
Protein helps balance your blood sugar and provides the necessary building blocks for brain health. And it's critically important throughout the aging process because it helps you maintain your lean muscle mass, a real issue as we age. Great sources of protein include fish, skinless turkey or chicken, beans, raw nuts, and high-protein vegetables such as broccoli and spinach. I use

spinach instead of lettuce in my salads for a huge nutrition boost. Protein powders can also be a good source, but read the labels. Many companies put a lot of sugar and other unhealthy ingredients in their powders. It is important to start each day with protein to boost your focus and concentration skills. More on this in a bit.

Rule 4. Eat Smart (Low-Glycemic, High-Fiber) Carbohydrates—Eat carbohydrates that do not spike your blood sugar and that are also high in fiber, such as those found in vegetables and fruits such as blueberries and apples. Carbohydrates per se are not the enemy. They are essential to your life. But bad carbohydrates *are* the enemy. These are carbohydrates that have been stripped of any nutritional value, such as simple sugars and refined carbohydrates. If you want to live without cravings, eliminate them completely from your diet. I like the saying "The whiter the bread the faster you are dead."

Sugar is *not* your friend. Sugar increases inflammation in your body, increases erratic brain cell firing, is addictive, and has been implicated in aggression. In a new study, children who were given sugar every day had a significantly higher risk for violence later in life. I don't agree with the people who say everything in moderation. Cocaine or arsenic in moderation is not a good idea. The less sugar in your life, the better your life will be, period.

Get to know the glycemic index. The glycemic index (GI) rates carbohydrates according to their effects on blood sugar. It is ranked on a scale from 1 to 100-plus (glucose is 100) with the low-glycemic foods having a lower number (which means they do not spike your blood sugar, so they are generally healthier for you) and the high-glycemic foods having a high number (which means they quickly elevate your blood sugar, so they are generally not as healthy for you). In general, I like to stay under 60.

Eating a diet that is filled with low-glycemic foods will lower your blood glucose levels, decrease cravings, and help with weight loss. The important concept to remember is that high blood sugar levels are bad for your blood vessels, brain, and your waistline.

However, you'll want to be careful not to go only by the GI to choose your foods. Some low-glycemic foods aren't healthy for you. For example, peanut M&Ms have a GI of 33, whereas steel-cut oatmeal has a GI of about 52. Does this mean that it's better for you to eat peanut M&Ms? No! Peanut M&Ms are loaded with saturated fat, artificial food coloring, and other things that are not good for your brain. Steel-cut oatmeal is a high-fiber food that helps regulate your blood sugar for hours. Use your brain when choosing your food.

In general, vegetables, fruits, legumes, and nuts are the best low-GI options. A diet rich in whole, minimally processed low-GI foods not only helps you lose weight; it has also been found to help control diabetes, according to a 2010 review of the scientific literature in the *British Journal of Nutrition*. Be aware, however, that some foods that sound healthy actually have a high GI. For example, some fruits like watermelon and pineapple have a high ranking. It is wise to consume more fruits on the low end of the spectrum. Similarly, some starches like potatoes and some high-fiber products like whole wheat bread are on the high end of the list. Eating smaller portions of these foods, thinking of them more like a condiment, and combining them with lean proteins and healthy fats can reduce their impact on blood sugar levels.

 View the Glycemic Index of many foods

Choose high-fiber carbohydrates. High-fiber foods are one of your best weight-loss weapons. Years of research have found that the more fiber you eat, the better for your health and weight. How does dietary fiber fight fat?

First, it helps regulate the appetite hormone ghrelin, which tells your brain that you are hungry. Ghrelin levels are often out of balance in people with a high BMI, so they always feel hungry, no matter how much they eat. New research shows that high ghrelin levels not only make you feel hungrier, they also increase the desire for high-calorie foods compared to low-calorie fare, so it's a double whammy. But fiber can help. A 2009 study showed that eating a diet high in fiber helped balance ghrelin levels in overweight and obese people. This can turn off the constant hunger and reduce the appeal of high-calorie foods.

Second, no matter how much you weigh, eating fiber-rich foods helps you feel full longer, ensuring that you don't get the munchies an hour after you eat.

Third, fiber slows the absorption of food into the bloodstream, which helps balance your blood sugar. This can help you make better food choices and fight cravings later in the day. In fact, fiber takes so long to be digested by your body, a person eating a diet that provides 20–35 grams of fiber a day will burn an extra 150 calories a day and lose 16 extra pounds a year.

These three things alone can go a long way in helping you avoid extra calories. Fiber-friendly foods boast a number of other health benefits as well, including:

- Reducing cholesterol
- Keeping your digestive tract moving
- Reducing high blood pressure
- Reducing the risk of cancer

Experts recommend eating 25–35 grams of fiber a day, but research shows that most adults fall far short of that. So how can you boost your fiber intake? Eat more high-fiber brain-healthy foods like fruits, vegetables, and legumes. Here is a link to the fiber contents of some brain-healthy foods. Try to include some of the foods on this list at every meal or snack.

View the fiber content of brain-healthy foods

Rule 5. Focus Your Diet on Healthy Fats—Fat is not the enemy. Good fats are essential to your health. The solid weight of your brain, after all the water is removed is 60 percent fat. When the medical establishment recommended we get fat out of our diets, we got fat. Bad fats are the enemy and you want to eliminate them, such as all trans fats. Did you know that certain fats that are found in pizza, ice cream, and cheeseburgers fool the brain into ignoring the signals that you should be full? No wonder I used to always eat two bowls of ice cream and eight slices of pizza. Focus your diet on healthy fats, especially those that contain omega-3 fatty acids, found in foods like salmon, avocados, walnuts, and green leafy vegetables.

High cholesterol levels are not good for your brain. A new study reports that people who had high cholesterol levels in their forties have a higher risk of getting Alzheimer's disease in their sixties and seventies. There is very good scientific evidence that the B vitamin niacin helps lower cholesterol and raise the level of HDL, the good cholesterol. Avocados and garlic can help as well. But don't let your cholesterol levels go too low. Low cholesterol levels have been associated with both homicide and suicide. If I am at a party and someone is bragging to me about their low cholesterol levels, I am always *very* nice to that person.

 View a list of foods high in omega-3 fatty acids

Rule 6. Eat Natural Foods of Many Different Colors—This means you should eat foods from all the colors of the rainbow, such as blueberries, pomegranates, yellow squash, and red bell peppers. This will boost the antioxidant levels in your body and help keep your brain young. Of course, these rainbow colors do not include Skittles, jelly beans, or M&Ms.

 View a list of high antioxidant foods

Rule 7. Cook with Brain-Healthy Herbs and Spices to Boost Your Brain—Here is a little food for thought, literally.

- Turmeric, found in curry, contains a chemical that has been shown to decrease the plaques in the brain thought to be responsible for Alzheimer's disease.
- In three studies, a saffron extract was found to be as effective as antidepressant medication in treating people with major depression.
- There is good scientific evidence that indicates rosemary, thyme, and sage help boost memory.
- Cinnamon has been shown to help attention and blood sugar. It is high in antioxidants and is a natural aphrodisiac.

- Garlic and oregano boost blood flow to the brain.
- Ginger, cayenne, black pepper—the hot spicy taste comes from gingerols, capsaicin, and piperine, compounds that boost metabolism and have an aphrodisiac effect.

Rule 8. Make sure your food is as clean as possible—As much as possible, eat organically grown foods, as pesticides used in commercial farming can accumulate in your brain and body, even though the levels in each food may be low. Also, eat meat that is hormone- and antibiotic-free; animals from which meat comes from should be free range and grass-fed. It is critical to know and understand what the foods you eat ate. In addition, eliminate food additives, preservatives, and artificial dyes and sweeteners. This means you must start reading the labels. If you do not know what is in something, do not eat it. Would you ever spend money on something if you did not know the cost of it? Of course not. Now is the time to really get thoughtful and serious about the food you put in your body.

Fourteen Foods with the Highest Levels of Pesticide Residues (Buy Organic)
1. Celery
2. Peaches
3. Strawberries
4. Apples
5. Blueberries
6. Nectarines
7. Cucumbers
8. Bell peppers
9. Spinach

10. Cherries
11. Collard greens and kale
12. Potatoes
13. Grapes
14. Green beans

Seventeen Foods with the Lowest Levels of Pesticide Residues
1. Onions
2. Avocados
3. Sweet corn (frozen)
4. Pineapples
5. Mangoes
6. Asparagus
7. English sweet peas (frozen)
8. Kiwi fruit
9. Bananas
10. Cabbage
11. Broccoli
12. Papaya
13. Mushrooms
14. Watermelon
15. Grapefruit
16. Eggplant
17. Cantaloupe

Fish is a great source of healthy protein and fat, but it is important to consider the toxicity in some fish. Here are a couple of general rules to guide you: (1) The larger the fish, the more mercury it may contain, so go for the smaller varieties. (2) From the safe fish choices, eat a fairly wide variety of fish, preferably those highest in omega-3s, like wild Alaskan salmon, anchovies, and Pacific halibut.

View a list of eco-friendly fish

Rule 9. If You're Having Trouble with Your Mood, Energy, Memory, Weight, Blood Sugar, Blood Pressure, or Skin, Eliminate Any Foods That Might Be Causing Trouble, Especially Wheat and Any Other Gluten-Containing Grain or Food, Dairy, Soy, and Corn—Did you know that gluten can literally make some people crazy? There are scientific reports of people having psychotic episodes when they're exposed to gluten, and when they eliminate wheat and other gluten sources (such as barley, rye, spelt, imitation meats, soy sauce) from their diets, their stomachs and their brains are better. One of my patients lost 30 pounds, and her moodiness, eczema, and irritable bowel symptoms completely went away when she got wheat out of her diet. Another one of my patients would become violent whenever he ate MSG. When we scanned him on MSG his brain changed into a pattern more consistent with our aggressive patients.

Autistic children and children with attention deficit hyperactivity disorder (ADHD) often do better when we put them on elimination diets that get rid of wheat, dairy, all the processed foods, food dyes, and additives.

There are blood tests you can take to learn more about your sensitivities to food. In addition, go to this link to try the Food Elimination diet we use at the Amen Clinics.

View instructions for the food elimination diet

THE AMEN CLINICS NINE RULES OF
BRAIN-HEALTHY EATING

1. Rule 1. Think "high-quality calories" but not too many of them.

2. Rule 2. Drink plenty of water and avoid liquid calories.

3. Rule 3. Eat high-quality lean protein throughout the day.

4. Rule 4. Eat smart (low-glycemic, high-fiber) carbohydrates.

5. Rule 5. Focus your diet on healthy fats.

6. Rule 6. Eat natural foods of many different colors.

7. Rule 7. Cook with brain-healthy herbs and spices to boost your brain.

8. Rule 8. Make sure your food is as clean as possible.

9. Rule 9. If you're having trouble with your mood, energy, memory, weight, blood sugar, blood pressure, or skin make sure to eliminate any foods that might be causing trouble, especially wheat and any other gluten containing grain or food, dairy, soy, and corn.

Fifty-two Best Brain-Healthy Superfoods That Can Help You Unleash the Power of the Female Brain

To help you get started on the right path, here is my list of the fifty-two best brain-healthy superfoods for the female brain based on the above principles. Make sure these foods are organic and, when appropriate, hormone- and antibiotic-free; animals should be free range and grass-fed.

Nuts and Seeds

1. Almonds, raw—for protein, healthy fats, and fiber

2. Brazil nuts—great source of zinc, magnesium, thiamine, high selenium content, healthy fat, and fiber

3. Cacao, raw—loaded with antioxidants, high in flavonoids, substances shown to increase blood flow, magnesium, iron, chromium, zinc, copper, and fiber. Can help decrease cravings and balance blood sugar, and it can make you happy by stimulating both serotonin, endorphins, and phenylethylamine.

But eat only a small amount of dark chocolate or it will turn into fat.

4. Cashews—rich in phosphorus, magnesium, zinc, and anti-oxidants
5. Chia seeds—very high in plant-based omega-3 fatty acids, fiber, and antioxidants
6. Coconut—high in fiber, manganese, and iron; low in natural sugars; high in medium-chain triglycerides shown to be helpful for brain tissue
7. Hemp seeds—high in protein, contain all essential amino acids and fatty acids, high in omega-3s and healthy omega-6s, including 6-gamma-linolenic acid, which has anti-inflammatory properties; also high in fiber and vitamin E
8. Sesame seeds—high in fiber, help stabilize blood sugar and lower cholesterol; good source of calcium, phosphorous, and zinc
9. Walnuts—of all nuts, contain the most omega-3 fatty acids to help lower bad cholesterol and may reduce inflammation; great source of antioxidants, vitamin E, selenium, and magnesium

Legumes (small amounts)
10. Chickpeas—for their high serotonin content
11. Lentils—for fiber

Fruits
12. Acai berries—for fiber, omega-3s, antioxidants, minerals, vitamins, plant sterols, and phytonutrients; low GI and sugar
13. Apples—rich in antioxidants and fiber; will help you not overeat
14. Avocados—high in omega-3 fats, high in lutein (good for eyesight), and potassium and folate; low in pesticides

15. Blackberries—high in antioxidants, phytonutrients, and fiber; low GI

16. Blueberries—loaded with antioxidants. Anthocyanins, compounds that give blueberries their deep color, may have antidiabetic effects. Some studies suggest these "brain berries" may help make you smarter

17. Cherries—high in fiber, low GI

18. Goldenberry—high in fiber, phosphorous, calcium, and vitamins A, C, B_1, B_2, B_6, and B_{12}; very high in protein for fruit (16%)

19. Gogi berries—rich in antioxidants, fiber, amino acids, iron, and vitamin C; helps lower blood pressure, stabilize blood sugar, and fights yeast

20. Grapefruit—for fiber, nutrients, and lower GI

21. Honey, raw, wild (small amounts only)—rich in minerals, antioxidants, probiotics, all twenty-two essential amino acids. Some types from Hawaii (Lehua and Noni) and New Zealand (Manuka) have antifungal, antibacterial, and antiviral properties

22. Kiwi—for fiber, nutrients, and lower GI

23. Pomegranates—high in fiber and antioxidants; low in calories

Vegetables

24. Asparagus—for fiber and antioxidants

25. Beets—high in fiber, phytonutrients, folate, and beta carotene

26. Bell peppers—for fiber and vitamin C

27. Broccoli—cruciferous vegetable; loaded with sulforaphanes; may increase enzymes that lower the incidence of some cancers

28. Brussels sprouts—high in fiber; cruciferous vegetable; high in sulforaphanes; may increase enzymes that lower the incidence of some cancers

29. Cabbage—cruciferous vegetable; loaded with sulforaphanes; may increase enzymes that lower the incidence of some cancers

30. Cauliflower—cruciferous vegetable; loaded with sulforaphanes; may increase enzymes that lower the incidence of some cancers

31. Chlorella—blue-green algae; rich in chlorophyll; helps detoxify the body and remove dioxin, lead, and mercury; contains high concentrations of B vitamins and helps digestion.

32. Garlic—Allium botanical family; can help lower blood pressure and cholesterol; inhibits growth of some cancer; has antibiotic properties; boosts blood flow to the brain

33. Horseradish—high in calcium, potassium, vitamin C; helps maintain collagen

34. Kale and other dark leafy greens—contain omega-3 fats, iron (especially important for women), and phytonutrients

35. Leeks—Allium botanical family; can help lower blood pressure and cholesterol; inhibits growth of some cancer; has antibiotic properties

36. Maca root—South American root; extraordinarily rich in amino acids, minerals, plant sterols, vitamins, and healthy fatty acids

37. Onions—Allium botanical family; can help lower blood pressure and cholesterol; inhibits growth of some cancer; has antibiotic properties; boosts blood flow to the brain

38. Seaweeds—high in omega-3s and in magnesium

39. Spinach and other dark leafy greens—contain omega-3 fats, iron (especially important for women), and phytonutrients

40. Spirulina—highest concentration of any protein and a top source of iron (should not be eaten if your iron is too high); rich in antioxidants and can help you have healthy hair and skin

41. Sweet potatoes—loaded with phytonutrients, fiber, and vitamin A
42. Wheatgrass juice—dense with minerals and vitamins; contains 70 percent chlorophyll; complete protein with thirty enzymes; excellent source of phosphorus, magnesium, zinc, and potassium

Oils

43. Coconut oil—stable at high temperatures
44. Grapeseed oil—stable at high temperatures; high in omega-3s
45. Olive oil—stable only at room temperature

Poultry/Fish

46. Chicken or turkey, skinless —for low-fat protein
47. Eggs—for protein
48. Lamb—high in omega-3s
49. Salmon, wild—loaded with brain-boosting omega-3s
50. Sardines, wild caught—low in mercury, high in brain-boosting omega-3s, vitamin D, and calcium; sustainable.

Tea

51. Tea, preferably green—contains protective antioxidants, less caffeine than coffee, and metabolism-boosting compound epigallocatechin gallate; also contains theanine which helps you relax and focus at the same time

Special Category

52. Shiratake noodles (from the root of a wild yam plant); goes by brand name Miracle Noodles—high in fiber and low in calories; one of my wife's secret replacements for pasta

How to Control Your Mind and Mood with Food

Most people don't know that they can use food to manipulate their minds. Food can help you feel relaxed, happy, and focused, or downright dumb. How we feed ourselves and our children in this country is backward.

Generally, simple carbohydrates, such as those found in pancakes, waffles, muffins, bagels, or cereal, boost serotonin levels, which help us feel relaxed, calm, and less worried and motivated. Protein, found in meat, nuts, or eggs, boosts dopamine levels and helps us feel more driven, motivated, and focused. Yet many people eat simple carbs in the morning and have more protein-based meals at night.

For example, it is very common to feed children (and ourselves) a breakfast of doughnuts, pancakes, waffles, sugary cereals, muffins, bagels, or toast, along with fruit juices (concentrated sugar). Then we ask our children to focus, which can cause real problems and make them look like they have ADD (attention deficit disorder). These simple carbohydrate-based meals spike insulin, which can often cause low blood sugar levels in a short period of time, causing brain fog. In addition, simple carbohydrates spike serotonin levels in the brain, so we feel happier after the meal. The problem is that serotonin also can decrease our ability to get things done; it gives many people "don't worry, be happy" attitude. Not exactly the best mind-set for school or work. Protein-based meals tend to do the opposite. They can boost dopamine levels in the brain, give us energy, and help us focus.

Therefore, it makes sense to eat a protein-rich meal at the start of the day—or at dinner if you still need to get work finished in the evening. If you want to relax in the evening and go to bed early, I recommend decreasing the protein and eating more healthy carbohydrate-rich foods.

Often, when kids come home from school, parents give them a few cookies and a soda (a high- and simple-carbohydrate-based snack). Then they tell them to do their homework. Unfortunately, the parents have unwittingly diminished their children's ability to get their homework finished, and it causes a night of stress for everyone.

Foods to Boost Mood, Focus, Motivation, and Memory

As a reminder, serotonin is a neurotransmitter that helps soothe the brain. It is intimately involved in sleep, mood regulation, appetite, and social engagement. It helps decrease our worries and concerns. Based on research at MIT, foods rich in simple carbohydrates have been found to quickly boost serotonin. They cause a spike in insulin, which lowers most large amino acids with the exception of tryptophan, the amino acid building block for serotonin, thereby decreasing the competition for tryptophan to get into the brain. This is why many people can become dependent on or even addicted to bread, pasta, potatoes, rice, and sugar. They use these as "mood foods" and feel more relaxed and less worried after they eat them. Unfortunately, because they boost serotonin, they can also lower PFC function and diminish a person's internal braking ability. I think this is precisely why restaurants serve bread and alcohol before a meal. If you consume them, you are much more likely to order dessert.

Brain-healthy foods that help to boost serotonin include smart carbohydrates such as sweet potatoes, apples, blueberries, carrots, steel-cut oatmeal, and chickpeas. These cause a more gradual increase in serotonin. It is a myth that foods that contain high levels of tryptophan, such as turkey, actually raise serotonin in the brain. Tryptophan is transported into the brain by a system that is geared toward larger protein molecules, and tryptophan, being smaller and less abundant, doesn't compete well against the other proteins to get in the brain. This is one of the main reasons that exercise helps people feel better. Exercise pushes the larger amino acids into your muscles and thereby decreases the competition for tryptophan to get into the brain. If you want to feel happier, grab an apple and go for a walk.

Dopamine is the neurotransmitter involved motivation, emotional significance, relevance, focus, and pleasure. It helps you get things done. Protein generally helps boost dopamine levels, which is why if you need to focus, avoid sugar, bread, pasta, rice, and white potatoes. Foods that tend to increase dopamine include beef, poultry, fish, eggs, seeds (pumpkin and sesame), nuts (almonds and walnuts), cheese, protein powders, and green tea. In addition, avocados and lima beans can help. Tyrosine is the amino acid building block for dopamine and is also essential for thyroid function. Simple carbohydrates tend to deplete dopamine.

Acetylcholine is the neurotransmitter involved with learning and memory. Liver, eggs, milk, salmon, and shrimp tend to boost these levels.

Heal Your Gut to Boost Your Brain

The gut is often called the second brain. It is loaded with nervous tissue and is in direct communication with our big brain, which is why we get butterflies when excited or have loose bowels when upset. Anxiety, depression, stress, and grief all express themselves with emotional pain (the brain) and quite often gastrointestinal distress.

Your gut is one of the most important organs for the health of your female brain. It is estimated that the gastrointestinal tract is loaded with about one hundred trillion microorganisms (bacteria, yeast, and others), about ten times the total number of cells in the human body. To be healthy, the relationship of good bugs to bad bugs needs to be lopsided in the positive direction, around 85 percent good guys to 15 percent bad guys. When it goes the other way and the bad bugs get a foothold, all sorts of physical and mental problems can arise. Keeping the good and bad bugs in proper balance is essential to your mental health.

There is new evidence that friendly gut bacteria actually deter invading troublemakers, such as *E. coli,* and help us withstand stress. If the friendly bugs are deficient, either from a poor diet that feeds yeast overgrowth (think sugar), or the excessive use of antibiotics (even as far back as childhood) that killed the good bacteria, we are more likely to feel stressed. Disorders ranging from ADD to autism in children, and depression to mental fogginess in adults, have been connected to intestinal bacteria imbalances that cause increased gut permeability.

The intestines provide an important barrier to bad bugs from the outside world. If they become too permeable, a condition referred to as leaky gut, inflammation and illness can be created throughout the body. Optimizing the "gut–brain axis" is critical to your mental health.

Factors That Decrease Healthy Gut Bacteria
- Medications (antibiotics, oral contraceptives, proton pump inhibitors, steroids, NSAIDs)
- Refined sugar intake
- Artificial sweeteners
- Bactericidal chemicals in water
- Pesticide residues in food
- Alcohol
- Physiological, emotional, and environmental stressors
- Radiation
- High-intensity exercise

The greatest danger from antibiotics does not come from those prescribed by your doctor but rather from the foods you eat. The prevalence of antibiotics found in conventionally raised meats and vegetables have the potential to throw off the balance of good to bad bacteria. It is estimated that 70 percent of the total antibiotic use in the United States is for livestock. It is critical to focus on eating antibiotic-free, hormone-free meats from grass-fed, free-range animals.

A Few Good Germs Can Be Good for You

Animals raised in a germ-free environment show exaggerated responses to psychological stress. We all need the good bugs in our intestinal tract to boost our immune system, so be careful not to go overboard in keeping your children away from the dirt. When researchers gave the animals probiotics (healthy bugs), their stress levels normalized.

Stress, all by itself, decreases healthy gut flora. Early abandonment issues can cause increased stress, decreased healthy bacteria, and increased gut permeability. When young rats were separated from their mothers, the layer of cells that line the gut became more permeable, allowing bacteria from the intestine to pass through the bowel walls and stimulate immune cells to start attacking other organs. "In rats, it's an adaptive response," reports Dr. Emeran Mayer from UCLA. "If they're born into a stressful, hostile environment, nature programs them to be more vigilant and stress responsive in their future life." Dr. Mayer said that up to 70 percent of the patients he treats for chronic gut disorders had experienced early childhood traumas like parents' divorces, chronic illnesses, or parents' deaths. "I think that what happens in early life, along with an individual's genetic background, programs how a person will respond to stress for the rest of his or her life."

Teresa grew up in a single-parent home filled with stress. At the age of four, her uncle was murdered, and shortly thereafter her mother brought Teresa to the doctor for gastrointestinal complaints. At age nine, Teresa started having panic attacks, especially when her mother came home late from work. As a teenager, she developed bulimia, again with bad intestinal issues. Decreasing her stress, along with giving her probiotics to help boost the friendly bugs in her gut, made a positive difference for her physically and emotionally.

In a recent study, Drs. A. Venket Rao and Alison Bested, administered thirty-nine patients with chronic fatigue syndrome either three doses of a probiotic (healthy bugs) a day or a placebo for two months. They found that 73 percent of subjects taking the probiotic experienced an increase in levels of good bacteria in the gut, which corresponded with a significant decrease in anxiety symptoms. The researchers found no significant change in anxiety for the placebo group. The researchers believed that probiotics "crowd out" the more toxic gut bacteria linked to depression and other mood disorders. Dr. Bested reported, "The subjects felt less anxious, calmer, better able to cope with their illness, sleeping better, had fewer heart palpitations, and less symptoms of anxiety."

What does this mean for you? Follow the brain-healthy food guidelines in this chapter carefully, especially by eliminating most of the simple sugars from your diet that feed the bad bugs. Focus on eating smart (low-glycemic, high-fiber) carbohydrates, which foster healthy flora. Also, consider taking a daily probiotic to give the good bugs a head start. Be careful with antibiotics. If you've had to take a lot of them in the past, a probiotic and healthy diet becomes even more important to the health of your brain.

PSYCHOLOGY

To get your food under control, it is critical to have the right thoughts and attitude about it. Getting healthy is about abundance, not deprivation. This is a critical mind shift to make. Being unhealthy or overweight is a thinking disorder, as much as it is an eating disorder. Many women refuse to get well because they cannot stand the idea of depriving themselves.

Once while I was doing consulting work for a large organization, the wife of the CEO told me that when we first introduced the brain-healthy program into the organization, she told her husband she would rather get cancer than give up sugar. That was when she realized that she had a serious problem with sugar.

Eating in a brain-healthy way is one of the strongest forms of self-love. If you truly love and care for yourself, you'll need to be diligent about putting only healthy fuel inside your body. But it takes the right thoughts and attitudes to make it happen. If you want to unleash the full power of your female brain, you have to be a warrior for the health of your brain.

Getting Your Thoughts Right About Food

How you think dramatically affects how you feel and *every decision you make*. And the lies you tell yourself are one of the biggest factors that drive illness. Here are some of the common "little lies" I hear about food.

- "I don't want to deprive myself." Doesn't eating bad food deprive you of your health, your most precious resource? What is worth more—energy, a trim waistline, and health, or the mountain of fries, sodas, cakes, cookies, and the like you have consumed over the last decade?
- "I can't eat healthy because I travel." I am always amused by this one, because I travel a lot. It just takes a little forethought and planning.
- "My whole family is overweight, so it's in my genes." This is one of the biggest lies. Genes account for only 20–30% of your health. The vast majority of health problems are driven by the bad decisions you make. My genes say I'm likely to be fat, but I make the decisions to ensure that it will be less likely to happen.
- "I can't afford to get healthy." Being sick is always more expensive than getting healthy.
- "I can't find the time to work out." With a sharper mind that comes from exercising, you will find that working out ultimately saves you time.
- "Not today—it's Easter, Memorial Day, Fourth of July, Labor Day, Thanksgiving, Christmas, Monday, Tuesday, Wednesday, Thursday, Friday, Saturday, or Sunday." There is always an excuse to hurt yourself.

When you stop believing every thought you have, the quality of your decisions and your health will go way up. So what are the lies you are telling yourself about food? Write them down now. In the next chapter, I'll teach ways to talk back to them,

How to Break the Hurtful Psychological Food Patterns from the Past

In a therapy session, Nancy-Lynn, a fifty-five-year-old woman who was working on getting healthy, told me she felt sad because she would not be able to bake with her grandchildren. The time spent baking cookies, brownies, and cakes with her grandmother was one of the most treasured parts of her childhood. As I listened, I could see the patterns from the past and negative thinking trying to hijack her brain and progress.

"Let's play this out," I said. "You are feeling sad because it is not in your best interest to bake cookies with your granddaughters?"

"Yes," she replied.

"Why would you not bake cookies with them?"

"Well, for one, it would ruin my program. The smell of freshly baked cookies is too much too resist."

"Any other reason?"

"If I bake cookies with them, I am planting the seeds of illness in their minds, like my grandmother unknowingly did to me. Cookies and other baked goodies are mood foods for me. They totally remind me of my grandmother's love."

With a smile I replied, "I suppose if you don't bake cookies or cakes or other toxic foods with them, then there is no other option for spending high-quality time with them?"

"Dr. Amen that is one of the dumbest things I have ever heard you say. Of course, there are other things I can do with them. Actually, I am sitting here thinking I can teach them how to cook in healthy ways. They can help me make great smoothies, salads, guacamole, veggie trays, and low-glycemic fruit plates. I can give them a legacy of health that they can do with their grandchildren, and that way they won't have these toxic, stupid thoughts."

My patients often say the smartest things. I just have to ask the right questions. Observe the patterns from your past that you are having trouble letting go of. Do they serve you or do they hurt you? Nancy-Lynn's pattern clearly was not only hurting her but also those she loved most.

SOCIAL CONNECTIONS

Preparing meals and feeding families is an important social activity. Being Lebanese, I know about this firsthand. We are known for great-tasting Mediterranean food. It can be incredibly healthy (think hummus, tabouleh, and grilled fish or lamb); or incredibly unhealthy (think butter cookies and baklava). Throughout my life, it has been common for my mother, wife, aunts, sisters, daughters, and nieces to be in the kitchen together cooking great meals. When the mother leads the brain-health charge, she has a huge influence on those who follow. The earlier you start, the better.

Social ties are so strong that researchers have found that the health of our family and friends is one of the strongest predictors of longevity. In 1921, Stanford psychologist Lewis Terman evaluated 1,548 ten-year-old children. He and subsequent researchers then followed this group over the next ninety years looking for the traits that were associated with success, health, and longevity. One of the main findings of the research was that social relationships had a dramatic impact on health. If your friends and family were unhealthy, you were much more likely to be like them. For people who want to improve their health, associating with other healthy people is usually the strongest and most direct path to change.

This does not mean you have to give up all of your friends and family who are struggling with their health; share this program with them and offer to do it together.

Right now, I want you to think of the people you love most in this world. Who do you call when something good—or bad—happens?

For me, I call my wife, my parents, and my children. For each of these people, ask yourself, "Am I their friend or their accomplice?" A friend is someone who helps their loved ones be successful; an accomplice is someone who helps them maintain their bad habits.

- "Oh, come on, it will be fine—it's just one time."
- "I cooked for you all weekend. Have more."
- "Don't be a party pooper."
- "It's the weekend—you've worked hard, so you've earned it."

Are you helping those you love prevent devastating illnesses like Alzheimer's and depression? Or are you unknowingly encouraging them to be sick? You can lead the change in your family.

SPIRITUAL HEALTH (SOUL FOOD)

Your sense of spirituality underlies everything you do. As we have discussed, it is the fuel that provides your life with a deep sense of meaning, passion, and purpose; it is your connection to God, past generations, future generations, and the future of our planet. In regard to food, ask yourself, "What is the underlying meaning and purpose for the food I eat and feed my family?" Is it just for basic nutrition? For pleasure? Fellowship? Is it to sustain my life so I can accomplish why I am here on Earth?" If your life has meaning and purpose, it is best served by a highly nutritious diet that nourishes your brain, body, and soul.

When I was first asked to a be a consultant for the Daniel Plan, Saddleback Church's plan for using religious organizations to get the world healthy, Pastor Rick Warren talked about the biblical directive to honor our bodies: "Do you not know that your body is a temple of the Holy Spirit, who is in you, whom you have received from God? You are not your own; you were bought at a price. Therefore honor God with your body" (1 Cor. 6:19–20). The way many people eat is definitely not honoring their bodies.

I like to use the acronym SOUL food to describe how to eat in a spiritual way. It stands for:

- Sustainable. We can continue to grow the food indefinitely without hurting our planet.
- Organic. Our food is raised in a clean environment without toxins.
- Unadulterated. We eat pure whole foods, without artificial food dyes, sweeteners, or additives.
- Locally grown. Our food is fresh, and we can support our local community by purchasing it.

From a spiritual standpoint, think about how the food you ingest was raised. If you eat meat, make it a point to know what the animals were fed, because you are also consuming what they ate. Also, think about how the animals were raised and harvested. Is it humane? Would it make you sick if you knew? If you think of eating as a spiritual discipline, these are essential questions.

One thought that has concerned me for a long time is how animals are raised and harvested. Animals, like humans, release different chemicals in their bodies when they feel relaxed or stressed, happy or depressed, approachable or angry. If they are raised and then killed in a confined, toxic environment in which they feel stressed, angry, and depressed, then ultimately we are consuming the chemicals the animals released when they were stressed, angry, and depressed. How your food was treated matters to the health of your body.

Eating as a spiritual discipline will help you not only give thanks for the food you have but also take a much more thoughtful approach to raising, harvesting, and consuming it.

Hour 5 Exercise—Provide Therapy for Your Kitchen

Just as therapists explore the cabinets of your mind and help to clean them of the toxic memories, I want you to take an hour to clean out your kitchen of any unhealthy or toxic food. Refer to the nine rules of brain-healthy eating outlined in this chapter. If the food doesn't serve your health, get rid of it. Don't donate it to the poor. It will make them sick as well.

View a video of Tana and me cleaning out the kitchen cabinets

View a video of Tana and Dr. Hyman on how to shop

6

SOOTHE THE FEMALE BRAIN

PUT AN END TO ANXIETY, WORRY, DEPRESSION, AND PERFECTIONISM

Calming and soothing your brain is the sixth step to unleashing the power of the female brain.
My mind perched on top of my head like a spider monkey and thought of more things that could go wrong. . . . My mind is my main problem almost all of the time. I wish I could leave it in the fridge when I go out, but it likes to come with me.

—ANNE LAMOTT

As discussed earlier, your female brain has many unique strengths, including intuition, empathy, collaboration, self-control, and a tendency to worry a little. But it is also important to recognize that it has some specific vulnerabilities. Consider the following facts:

- Females produce less serotonin than men, in one study by 52 percent. Although this likely helps them avoid the "don't worry, be happy" mind-set that gets many men in trouble, it can also set up women to have more problems with anxiety, depression, and worry.

- Estrogen inhibits the neurotransmitter GABA, which helps calm your brain, making females more likely to struggle with anxiety.
- Testosterone boosts GABA, which can lead males to feel less anxiety. When testosterone levels are high, in men or women with PCOS, it can lead to low levels of anxiety and high risk-taking behaviors.
- When female mice are given testosterone as adolescents, they are less likely to have depression as adults. This implies that adolescent girls should decrease their sugar intake (which lowers testosterone) and lift light weights to boost testosterone levels.
- Women, because of lower serotonin levels have busier brains, and they are more vulnerable to depression. Across many nations, cultures, and ethnicities, women are about twice as likely as men to be diagnosed with depression The lifetime incidence of major depression is 21.3 percent in women; it is 12.7 percent in men.
- Some researchers, however, believe that men experience depression in different ways than women, so they are not appropriately diagnosed. Instead of sadness, a man's depression is more likely to show up as anger, irritability, and recklessness. Plus, they are much less likely to seek help. A 2008 journal article titled "Women Seek Help, Men Die" highlights that men are four times more likely to kill themselves than women are. Seeking help is the strength of the female brain.
- Women respond better to a class of antidepressants called SSRIs.
- SSRIs do not work nearly as well in men, or when estrogen is not present in women, such as before puberty or after menopause.

- Men and postmenopausal women do better on more stimulating antidepressants, such as imipramine or buproprion.
- Over their lifetimes, women experience more major emotional traumas, particularly sexual abuse, than do men.
- With increased stress and trauma women are more likely to develop a heightened stress response, which is worsened during times of hormonal fluctuations (e.g., premenstrual, after delivering a baby, and during the transition phase to menopause).
- Anxiety disorders, including panic disorder, PTSD, social phobia, and generalized anxiety disorder, are more common in women.
- PTSD and substance abuse occur more commonly together in women. Getting sober may make PTSD symptoms worse in some women, as they lose their form of self-medication.
- Eating disorders are much more common in females than males.
- Addictions often progress more rapidly in women. Women are more sensitive to the euphoric effects of stimulants, such as amphetamine and cocaine.
- Female intelligence is more centralized in the brain's frontal lobes. Therefore, injuries to the frontal lobe can be more detrimental to cognitive performance in women than they are in men.
- Some studies report that Alzheimer's disease disproportionately affects women.

This chapter will help you develop a plan to overcome these vulnerabilities and help you feel better overall.

During the 2012 NBA playoffs, Tana and I went to a Lakers' game. At half-time, there was a female Chinese performer who was amazing.

The Staples Center was dark, except for a large spotlight on her. With long, jet black hair and a sparkling white pantsuit and hat, she rode out to center court on a unicycle. Her assistant put a white bowl upside down on her right foot, which she promptly flipped onto her head.

"Wow," I thought. "That takes skill."

There was mild applause from the distracted crowd, waiting for the game to resume. The assistant then placed two bowls on her left foot, and she did the same thing. Now she was balancing three bowls on her head. There was more applause and people were a bit more attentive. Then the assistant put three bowls in her right foot, and seemingly without any effort she flipped them onto the other three bowls on her head.

"My goodness," I thought.

Then the assistant placed four bowls on her left foot, and again she flipped all four bowls onto the other six. Ten bowls were now balanced on her head. The crowd roared with approval and were much more focused on the woman on the unicycle. Then the assistant put five bowls on each of her feet.

"No way," I said to Tana.

Yet she flipped the five bowls on one foot onto her head and then the other five bowls from the other foot. Now she was balancing twenty bowls on her head. The crowd jumped up and gave her a standing ovation, and she bowed, giving all twenty bowls to her assistant.

As I watched this amazing performance, I marveled at this woman's mastery. How many years of practice had gone into her ability to turn her body into an instrument of such skill? How much discipline was required to balance the unicycle and the bowls, where one wrong move might mean a dangerous fall or a serious injury? Her movements required physical control, yes, but they also represented years of mental and emotional control.

You are capable of this kind of emotional discipline and mastery. As we saw in chapter 2, a woman's busy brain can be a real advantage in many circumstances. But it can also lead you to feel overwhelmed by worries, sorrow, and stubborn thoughts you can't dismiss. Panic attacks, stress, suffering, and depression may be lessened or even completely resolved by learning specific techniques to train and discipline your brain.

Monkey mind is a Buddhist term for thoughts that run wild inside your skull. Here I will give you a clear roadmap to tame your monkey mind"; soothe your active brain; and decrease your risk of anxiety, depression, and eating disorders. Ultimately, they are all thinking disorders.

In my work with women, I have seen many apply the same kind of discipline and mastery to their mind as this performer applied to her body and achieve amazing results. Yes, it takes some consistent work, just as the performer had to do to achieve her amazing result. If you're going to be competent at anything, to achieve either physical or mental mastery, you have to practice. Yet the rewards are great.

Studies report that cognitive therapy—learning how to discipline your mind—is as effective, or in some studies even more effective, than antidepressant medications for anxiety, depression, and eating disorders. Better still, there are no bad side effects. Calm, clarity, flexibility, and a vastly improved mood are the immediate rewards for soothing your brain. Long-term results include a sense of calm, empowerment, and self-control.

MONKEY MIND UNLEASHED

You feel fat after eating too much, hate yourself, and make yourself throw up—and then hate yourself more.

Your boyfriend doesn't call when you expect him to, and you begin to worry that he's cheating on you or that he doesn't love you anymore. When he does call, you start to yell at him before he can explain what happened.

Your husband forgets your birthday *and* your anniversary, and you feel sad, neglected, and lonelier than you ever thought possible. When he comes home, you just ignore him, even though he asks again and again what you are upset about.

Your kids need to be picked up, your boss needs you to stay late for a new deadline, and your sister needs help with the family dinner she's planning. You feel frantic about getting everything done and making sure everyone's okay. Your heart is racing and you start to have diarrhea.

You think you are going to have a panic attack at the grocery store. You visualize fainting and the ambulance coming to take you to the hospital. Without processing the thought, you just leave your basket full of groceries and drive home.

Your widowed mother is getting older, and you are concerned that she can't live alone much longer. You start to feel overwhelmed with sadness.

Your sixteen-year-old daughter is just starting to date, and you worry about her making the same mistakes you made. Then you start to become very worried and forbid her from dating altogether, over her father's objections, which causes a big blowup.

You are single and worry that you will never find love, or perhaps you're in a relationship and feeling sad because it doesn't seem to be moving toward the commitment you would ideally like. You begin to feel frantic and upset during large chunks of the day.

You want to get healthy, but you hate the idea of giving up cake and cookies. You don't want to feel deprived. You feel sad and stuck either way you think, because you know you cannot get healthy eating them.

Often you feel that if you can't do everything right, you are a total failure and should just give up, but you can't give up, because too many people are counting on you.

Sometimes it feels like your mind is truly out of control.

Does any of this sound familiar? If so, you're not alone.

THE FOUR CIRCLES APPROACH TO DISCIPLINING YOUR MIND

To soothe your brain you need to get control over and discipline your mind. As we will see, you will have to turn your brain on in order to turn it off. Optimizing the four circles is the foundation of disciplining your mind.

BIOLOGY

To soothe your mind, it is critical to avoid anything that hurts your brain and to engage in regular brain-healthy habits. Also, make sure to get your important numbers and labs checked. If your thyroid, progesterone, or gut flora levels are off, the monkey-mind thoughts will screech wildly through the recesses of your brain. No amount of mental discipline will be fully effective.

In addition, it is critical to keep your blood sugar stable and to make sure you get at least seven hours of sleep each night. Low blood sugar levels or a lack of sleep are both associated with lower overall blood flow to the brain, which results in bad decision making and an inability to inhibit the thoughts that torture you. The PFC of the human brain serves in large part an inhibitory function. It helps to settle down your emotional brain. When the frontal lobes are low in activity or blood flow, they cannot quiet the noisy thoughts; as a result, you suffer. This is why it is also important treat ADD, which is often associated with low PFC activity (more on this in chapter 8), and to rehabilitate any past brain injuries that affected the PFC.

Know Your Brain Type

Among other things, my brain imaging work has taught me that knowing about your own specific brain type is critical to soothing your mind. Not everyone has the same brain.

When I first started to do our brain imaging work at the Amen Clinics in 1991, I was looking for the one pattern that was associated with anxiety, depression, addictions, or ADD. But I soon discovered there was clearly not one brain pattern associated with any of these illnesses. They all had multiple types. Of course, I then realized that there would never be just one pattern for depression, because not all depressed people are the same. Some are withdrawn; others are angry; still others are anxious or obsessive.

The scans helped me understand the type of anxiety, depression, ADD, obesity, or addiction a person had, so I could better target treatment to individual brains. This one idea led to a dramatic breakthrough in my own personal effectiveness with patients, and it opened up a new world of understanding and hope for the tens of thousands of people who have come to the Amen Clinics and the millions of people who have read my books. In previous books, I have written about six types of ADD, seven types of anxiety and depression, six types of addictions, and five types of overeaters. Understanding these types is critical to getting the right help.

Let me briefly review five of the brain types most important to soothing the female brain.

Brain Type 1: Impulsive—People with an impulsive brain type have poor impulse control, get distracted easily, and have trouble not saying or doing whatever comes into their minds. Typically the SPECT scans show low activity in the PFC. Think of the PFC as the brain's brake. It stops us from saying stupid things or making bad decisions. It is the little voice in your head that helps you decide between the banana and the banana split. The impulsive brain type is common among people who have ADD, which has been associated with low dopamine levels in the brain. People with ADD struggle with a short attention span, distractibility, disorganization, restlessness, and impulsivity. Think hyperactive monkey thoughts here. Without boosting the PFC, it is nearly impossible to get the monkeys under control.

My research team and I have published several studies showing that when people with the impulsive brain type try to concentrate, they actually get less activity in the PFC, which will cause them to have even less control over their own behavior. For these people, literally, the harder they try to lose weight the worse it gets. Smokers and heavy coffee drinkers also tend to fit this type.

This type is best helped by boosting dopamine levels in the brain to strengthen the PFC. Higher-protein, lower-carbohydrate diets tend to help, as does exercise and certain stimulating supplements, such as green tea, rhodiola, ginseng, or L-tyrosine, or medications, such as stimulants like Adderall or Concerta. In general, I am very cautious with medications, and they are usually not my first choice. Any supplement or medicine that calms the brain, such as 5-HTP or SSRIs, usually makes this type worse, because they lower PFC function and take the brakes off the brain. I have treated dozens of women who had done things that they later regretted, such as becoming hypersexual or spending money they did not have, when they were put on SSRIs. It turned out they had low activity in the PFC, and the serotonin-boosting medications diminished the judgment part of their brains.

Brain Type 2: Compulsive—People with a compulsive brain type tend to get stuck on negative thoughts or negative behaviors. They tend to worry and have trouble sleeping. In addition, they tend to be argumentative and oppositional and hold grudges from the past. People with this brain type generally have too much activity in the front part of the brain, in an area of the brain called the anterior cingulate gyrus, which functions as the brain's gear shifter. It gets sticky when there are low levels of a chemical called serotonin. When it is overactive, people can get stuck on the same thought. It is like having a little mouse on an exercise wheel in your head, and the mouse cannot get off. Thoughts tend to circle over and over and over.

Because caffeine and diet pills are stimulants, they tend to make this type worse, because this brain type does NOT need more stimulation, and women who have this type feel as though they may need a glass (or two or three) of wine at night to calm their worries. This type is associated with anxiety and depression. I have also seen it commonly in my patients with anorexia and obsessive-compulsive disorder.

The best strategy for calming this brain type is to find natural ways to boost serotonin, which is calming to the brain. Physical exercise boosts serotonin as do certain supplements, such as 5-HTP, inositol, saffron, and St. John's Wort. Medications that boost serotonin include the SSRIs, such as Prozac, Zoloft, Lexapro, Celexa, and Paxil.

Simple carbohydrates also increase serotonin, which is why many women become addicted to simple carbs like bread, pasta, and sugar. These are mood foods and are often used to self-medicate an underlying mood issue. Avoid these quick fixes as they help only in the short term but can cause long-term trouble.

Brain Type 3: Impulsive-Compulsive—On the surface, this brain type seems almost contradictory: How can someone be both impulsive and compulsive at the same time? Think of bulimia. People with an impulsive-compulsive brain type are compulsively driven to binge on food that is not healthy for them and yet have very little control over their impulses to binge or purge. It is the same with this type. Our scans tend to show too much activity in the anterior cingulate gyrus, the part of the brain that helps shift attention, so people overthink and get stuck on negative thoughts, but they also have too little activity in the PFC or impulsive control area, which means they have trouble supervising their own behavior.

In my experience, the impulsive-compulsive type is common in children and grandchildren of alcoholics.

People with this type benefit from treatments that increase both serotonin and dopamine, such as exercise with a combination of supplements like 5-HTP and green tea, or medications such as Prozac and Adderall. Using 5-HTP or green tea alone would make people with this type of brain worse.

Brain Type 4: SAD—The sad brain type is associated with frequent feelings of sadness, depression, low energy, low self-esteem, and pain symptoms. The SPECT scans tend to show too much activity in the limbic or emotional parts of the brain, which is common in mood disorders. For this type, boosting vitamin D can help, as can exercise, fish oil, supplements such as SAMe (S-adenosylmethionine), or medications such as Wellbutrin.

When women complain of depression to their primary care physicians, they are commonly prescribed an SSRI such as Prozac or Lexapro. In large-scale studies, these medications have as much chance of working as a placebo. The problem is not that these are not good medications; it is that depression is not any one kind, and one treatment will never work for all types of depression. In the sad brain type, the SSRIs tend to work if these women are also compulsive or overfocused. Absent those symptoms, however, these medications often make things worse.

Brain Type 5: Anxious—Anxiety, tension, nervousness, conflict avoidance, and a tendency to predict the worst are hallmarks of this anxious brain type. On SPECT, we often see too much activity in an area of the brain called the basal ganglia. This part of the brain is involved in setting a person's anxiety level. When there is too much activity here, owing to low levels of a chemical called GABA, people often have anxiety and a lot of physical tension.

Soothing this type with meditation and hypnosis, plus using a combination of B$_6$, magnesium, and GABA, our patients generally feel more relaxed and more in control of their minds. I avoid typical antianxiety medications, such as Xanax or Valium, as they have caused problems with addictions. If I need to use medications, I typically prescribe an anticonvulsant such as Neurontin to calm down excessive brain activity.

It is common to have more than one brain type. If that is true for you, work on the most bothersome brain type first and then move on to the others.

PSYCHOLOGY

Quieting and soothing your mind requires more than sleep, good blood sugar, probiotics, and targeted supplements for your brain type. It also requires practicing the habits of mental discipline and learning how to be honest with yourself. To help patients develop a disciplined mind, the Amen Clinics often teach the following psychological strategies: killing the ANTs, engaging in "the Work," and practicing hypnosis and meditation.

Killing the ANTs

One of the techniques that is the mainstay of helping our patients at the Amen Clinics is what I call ANT therapy, or learning how to kill the Automatic Negative Thoughts that you feel you have no control over. Learning how to not believe every stupid thought you have is a critical skill to ending the unnecessary suffering experienced by so many women. ANTs pop up in your brain automatically, seemingly out of nowhere, and when left unchallenged, they bite, nibble, torture, and infest your mind. When the ANTs are left unchecked, they steal your happiness and literally make you feel old, fat, depressed, and feebleminded.

The following exercise to kill the ANTS is so simple that you may have trouble believing how powerful it is, but I have seen it change many people's lives, including my own. Your suffering diminishes, and your health and happiness improve. A number of research studies have found this technique to be as effective and as powerful as antidepressant medication for anxiety, depression, and eating disorders.

ANT Therapy Directions

1. Whenever you feel sad, mad, nervous, or out of control, draw two lines vertically down a piece of paper, dividing it into three columns.

2. In the first column, write down the ANTs going through your mind.

3. In the second column, identify the type of ANT or negative thought. Therapists typically describe nine different types of ANTs (see the table on p. 000).

4. In the third column, talk back, correct, and eradicate the ANTs. If you were anything like me, you were good at talking back to your parents when you were a teenager. In the same way, you need to learn to be good at talking back to the lies you tell yourself.

ANT	ANT Type	ANT Killing
I will never be happy again.	Fortune-telling	I am sad now, but I will feel better soon.
I am a failure.	Labeling	I have succeeded at many things.
It is your fault!	Blame	I need to look at my part in the problem.
I should have done better.	Guilt beating	I will learn from my mistakes and do better next time.
I am old	Labeling	By working this program I can feel younger every day

In our online community (www.amensolution.com), you can do exercises to strengthen your ANT-killing abilities in our "Kill the ANTs" room. You can see examples and play therapeutic games to help you gain more skill at controlling and disciplining your mind.

View "Kill the ANTs"

SUMMARY OF NINE DIFFERENT TYPES OF ANTS

1. "Always" thinking: Overgeneralizing a situation; these thoughts usually start with words like *always, never, everyone,* and *every time*

2. Focusing on the negative: Focusing on what's going wrong in a situation and ignoring everything that could be construed as positive

3. Fortune-telling: Predicting the future in a negative way

4. Mind reading: Arbitrarily believing you know what another person thinks, even though they have not told you

5. Thinking with your feelings: Believing your negative feelings without ever questioning them.

6. Guilt beatings: Thinking in words like *should, must, ought,* or *have to*

7. Labeling: Attaching a negative label to yourself or others

8. Personalization: Construing innocuous events as having personal meaning

9. Blame: Blaming other people for the problems in your life

Empathy: A Blessing and a Curse

As we saw in chapter 2, empathy is a unique female strength. The downside to empathy is getting drawn into other people's sorrows and pain. That can lead you to become sad right along with them, as you take on their issues as if they were your own. You might also feel guilty about enjoying yourself and your own successes while people you care about are having a harder time. Many women feel guilty or anxious about making time and space for their own concerns, especially if a loved one is in trouble.

Any of us might be vulnerable to any of the ANTs. But empathy and a focus on your own emotions makes you prey to two ANTs in particular:

Thinking with Your Feelings—A key female strength is knowing what you're feeling. But the dark side of that strength is thinking with your feelings. For example, "I feel like you don't love me." Or "I feel like I'm being treated unfairly." Maybe you do feel that way, but is it true? Sometimes feelings lie, especially when you are tired, hungry, worried about something else, under a lot of stress, deprived of the brain chemicals you need, or struggling with a hormonal issue. Don't let your negative feelings rule your thoughts. Write them down and look for the evidence behind them.

Guilt Beatings—When you think in words like *should, must, ought,* or *have to,* you are likely beating yourself with guilt. I have heard this described as a "shower of shoulds." Women are often taught to put other people's needs first, so they feel guilty when they stand up for themselves or take time to de-stress. Guilt is frequently the result. I'm not saying you should ignore your own personal moral code. But see if you can reframe the guilt beatings into statements of what you truly want. Instead of "I *should* call up Casey and help her through her breakup," ask yourself if the behavior fits your goals and time. If the answer is no, call when it makes more sense for you. Having a process to free yourself from the guilt-beating ANTs will help settle down the noise in your head so you can make better choices.

Intuition: A Strength and a Weakness

Your female intuition enables you to see things that others miss and to know a great deal without being able to explain exactly how. Used correctly, your intuition can be an enormous strength. But it also opens you up to a great deal of worry and anxiety. If you believe your intuition without checking it out, you might end up "knowing" a lot that isn't true. Yes, sometimes you are right, but sometimes you've just invented your own reality, which is perhaps colored by lack of sleep, low blood sugar, or brain chemistry that has run amok. You run the risk of living in a world colored entirely by your own negative thoughts and free-floating feelings, which creates a lot of unnecessary anxiety and disrupted relationships. And you become prey to the fortune-telling and mind-reading ANTs.

> **Fortune-Telling**—When you engage in fortune-telling, you arbitrarily predict the worst ("I am going to fail this class"; "I'm going to have a panic attack in the grocery store"). When that happens, your heart beats faster, your breathing becomes faster and more shallow, and your adrenal glands start pumping out cortisol and adrenaline. Fortune-telling thoughts instantly push your stress levels higher. What's worse, predicting bad things can actually help them come true. If you are about to go on a date and you predict it won't go well, you'll focus on the first negative thing about the guy you can find, and then you will be less responsive, less cheerful, and less fun to be with. If you're sure that you'll have a bad day at work, you'll be in a terrible mood as soon as anything bad happens, and your day is certain to go downhill from there.
>
> **Mind Reading**—When you believe you know what someone else is thinking even though they have not told you, you are mind reading. If someone looks at you funny, you might think, "I know

she doesn't like me." That is mind reading. Maybe the person is just having a bad day! Drawing the line between your helpful intuition and the poisonous mind-reading ANT isn't always easy. But once you learn to kill this ANT, your relationships and mood will likely improve.

Collaboration or Codependence?

Collaboration is joining with another person in order to achieve a goal. That is usually a good thing and is a strength of the female brain. Collaboration has two dark sides, however. One is codependence, or the tendency to do for others what they should do for themselves, protecting them from the appropriate consequences of their own actions. The other is dependence: feeling that you can't do anything on your own without the permission or help of others. A tendency to either dependence or codependence can make it difficult for you to assert your own boundaries and maintain your own autonomy. You might end up feeling like a victim, which opens your mind to the personalization and "always" thinking ANTs.

> **Personalization**—A key female strength is building relationships, but the downside can be a tendency to personalize. "My husband didn't call; he must not love me anymore," is a classic example of personalization. Maybe the reason he didn't call has nothing to do with you: He's stressed, distracted, or dealing with a crisis. Another example is "My daughter at college failed her math test. I should have spent more time helping her with her homework in high school." Taking your daughter's failure personally is the act of an undisciplined mind, because by the time she's in college, your daughter's study habits should be her own responsibility, not yours. Neither blaming yourself for everything that goes wrong nor assuming that other people's actions are all about you are accurate reflections of reality. They're just ANTs.

"Always" Thinking—Any time you think in absolutes, usually characterized by such words as *always, never, no one, everyone, every time,* or *everything,* your negative thinking makes a temporary situation look like a permanent reality. Some examples: "He *never* listens to me." "I *always* have to do what she wants." "*Everyone* in this family gets their way except me." This kind of thinking closes your mind to other possibilities and keeps you focused on the negative, which will make you feel more anxious and/or depressed.

Focusing on the Negative—Most people and most experiences are a blend of positive and negative. It's important to use judgment wisely to avoid situations that are dangerous, abusive, unhealthy, or unpleasant, but it's also important not to take one negative element and blow it out of proportion. Since focusing on the negative almost always makes you feel bad, and focusing on the positive usually makes you feel better, a disciplined mind can focus on the positive while at the same time finding what is valuable in the negative. Where you bring your attention determines how you feel. I do not want you thinking in positive pie-in-the-sky happy thoughts just to feel good and ignore your health and well-being. I want you to be concerned when you need to be concerned, but also find the good in whatever situation you are in. An added benefit is that focusing on the positive opens you to a wider range of opportunities, which means that you are more likely to find people and situations that work out well for you.

Labeling—Attaching a negative label, whether to yourself or someone else, keeps you from taking a clear look at the person or situation that you labeled. "He's a jerk." "I'm an idiot." "What a stupid rule." "What an awful thing to say." Now instead of looking clearly at the specific person, rule, or comment, you are just lumping it in with all the other "jerks," "idiots," "stupid rules," and "awful remarks" you have known. Labeling won't necessarily help you deal with this particular issue, or to make accurate judgments about yourself. Avoid the labels and see things in their own terms.

Blame—Sometimes another person takes an action that hurts us. But even so, blame is very harmful. When we say, "If only you hadn't done *x,* I would have been all right," we are really saying, "You have all the power over my life, and I have none." The "blame game" undermines your sense of personal power. That is why it is the most poisonous ANT of all. Focus on what you can do about a situation and on what you want to do next, and don't allow those blaming ANTs any space in your mind.

Jenna: Stuck in a Rut

Jenna was a graphic designer in her mid-twenties who faced increasing trouble at her job. Although she had won several prestigious industry awards, she couldn't seem to get along with either her clients or her supervisor. She was frustrated at having to make compromises when she *knew* her opinion was correct, and she often found herself getting into arguments that she just couldn't seem to drop. She fought with her boyfriend too. "Once we start," she told me, "I just can't let it go. And then I remember every awful thing he ever did to me and I just go on the attack. I bring up stuff from three years ago, because it all feels like it just happened to me yesterday. It's like I get these thoughts into my head, and I just can't get them out."

Jenna was a classic case of the compulsive brain type. She got stuck on negative thoughts that she could not dislodge. Jenna found 5-HTP helpful to calm her overactive brain, along with exercise and a commitment to getting regular sleep. These biological approaches were not enough, however. Jenna also needed to learn how to kill her ANTs.

Jenna's most poisonous ANT was blame. Whenever anything bad happened to her, she tended to leap to the conclusion that someone else was to blame, rather than seeing how she had contributed to the situation, or at least viewing the situation from the perspective of others. I didn't want Jenna to shift from blaming others to blaming herself. But I did want her to stop feeling like a victim from her undisciplined her mind.

Here is how Jenna reframed her blame ANT:

> ANT: I'm having trouble meeting this deadline. It's because the client keeps changing his mind. I'm miserable, and it's all his fault!
>
> TYPE OF ANT: Blame
>
> KILLING THE ANT: I have chosen to do this work, which I mainly enjoy. Dealing with client requests and staying late to meet a deadline is part of the job. I'll make sure to build regular breaks into my schedule and to eat some healthy snacks so that I stay motivated and fresh while I complete this assignment.

> ANT: My boyfriend didn't call on time, and now it's too late to go to that movie I wanted to see. He's just ruined my night!
>
> TYPE OF ANT: Blame
>
> KILLING THE ANT: It's still early. Maybe I can go to a later show . . . or watch something on TV . . . or call a girlfriend and catch up with her on the phone. I don't have to give up all my fun for a whole evening just because of a missed phone call.

As Jenna disciplined her mind, she found an enormous side benefit: She no longer felt at the mercy of her own thoughts. Her thinking became more flexible, she felt calmer and less worried, and she began getting along better with her clients, co-workers, and loved ones. Disciplining her mind had allowed Jenna to soothe her brain, and her life worked better as a result.

Marley: Learning Not to be Perfect

Marley was a fifty-two-year-old single mother of three with a high-level job in the banking industry. Although she was highly successful at work and her children were doing fine, Marley worried constantly about what *might* go wrong. She often stayed awake for hours as her mind raced from one potential disaster to the next. Despite the many professional accolades she had received, Marley often felt like an impostor, and she frequently stayed late at the office to make sure her work was "perfect." When I looked at Marley, I saw a beautifully dressed woman with lovely clothes, impeccable hair, and bitten nails. While we talked, she picked at her cuticles, jiggled her leg, and looked as though she was going to jump right out of her chair. "I'm tired of always worrying about every little thing," she told me. "But I can't seem to stop."

Marley was a prime example of an intelligent, accomplished woman who nonetheless had an undisciplined mind and a busy brain. Because she always felt like an imposter or a fraud, she drove herself relentlessly to perfection, hoping that would prevent others from "seeing through her" and somehow undermining her position. Many women struggle with this problem, partly because they really do face opposition from both men and women at work, partly because they are prey to a number of ANTs.

Marley's worst ANTs were mind reading and personalization. She was constantly assuming that a co-worker didn't like her, an employee resented her direction, or a top executive was planning to get rid of her. She personalized company policies, seeing them as directed against her rather than understanding that they affected everyone and might have been instituted for reasons that had nothing to do with her. Her ANTs brought her a great deal of needless unhappiness, anxiety, and agitation.

Once I showed Marley how to kill her ANTs, she set about disciplining her mind with the same determination and energy that she had used to build her career in the first place. Here are the mental habits that Marley practiced every day to kill some of her ANTs:

ANT: She didn't smile at me when I walked by her desk, she must be mad about what I said to her in the meeting yesterday.

TYPE OF ANT: Mind reading

KILLING THE ANT: I have no way of knowing what it meant that she didn't smile. Maybe she didn't notice me. Maybe her child is sick. If I want to know what she's thinking, I have to ask her.

ANT: I was late three times last week when my daughter was sick—this new memo about lateness is obviously directed against me. I'd better make extra sure to come in on time, or I might not get a bonus this year.

TYPE OF ANT: Personalization

KILLING THE ANT: It's a big company, who knows why they sent this memo at this time. I'm one of twenty vice presidents. It seems *really* unlikely that my being a few minutes late would cause them to send out a company-wide memo. I'm doing a great job, and everyone knows it. My bonus is probably safe.

Adopting brain-healthy habits helped Marley soothe her brain, but it was also disciplining her mind that made a long-term difference. Although Marley told me that she had to work a lot at killing her ANTs, much like the performer mentioned at the beginning of the chapter had to work at her craft, she felt calmer, happier, and more empowered. As an extra bonus, her new sense of self-confidence actually improved her job performance, giving her even more reason to feel confident. Marley had seen that soothing her brain created a positive cycle to replace the vicious one. When she saw the great results she got, she knew they were worth all the discipline and hard work.

The Work: Another Technique

"The Work" is another ANT-killing technique that I teach all of my patients. It was developed by my friend Byron Katie and is explained in her book *Loving What Is*. Katie, as her friends call her, described her own experience suffering from suicidal depression. She was a young mother, businesswoman, and wife in the high desert of Southern California. She became severely depressed at the age of thirty-three. For ten years, she sank deeper and deeper into self-loathing, rage, and despair, with constant thoughts of suicide and paranoia. For the last two years, she was often unable to leave her bedroom and care for herself or her family. Then one morning in 1986, out of nowhere, Katie woke up in a state of amazement, transformed by the realization that when she believed her thoughts, she suffered, but when she questioned her thoughts, she didn't suffer.

Katie's great insight is that it is not life or other people that make us feel depressed, angry, stressed, abandoned, and despairing: It is our own thoughts that make us feel that way. In other words, we can live in a hell of our own making, or we can live in a heaven of our own making.

Katie developed a simple method of inquiry for questioning our thoughts. It consists of (1) writing down any of the thoughts that are torturing us, including any of those in which we are judging other people; (2) asking ourselves four questions, and (3) doing a turnaround. The goal is not positive thinking but rather accurate thinking. The four questions are:

1. Is this particular thought true?
2. Can I absolutely know that it's true?

3. How do I react when I believe that thought?

4. Who would I be without the thought? (Or how would I feel if I didn't have the thought?)

Turnaround—After you answer the four questions, you then take the original thought and completely turn it around to its opposite, and ask yourself whether the opposite of the original thought that is causing your suffering is not true or even truer than the original thought. Then take the turned-around thought and apply it to yourself (and to the other person, if someone else is involved in the thought).

In my office I frequently find myself at my white board, writing these four questions as a way to help people talk back to the thoughts that make them suffer.

Celeste, forty-eight, was a divorced mother of eight children. She came to me after being unable to shake feelings of depression and inadequacy. Since her divorce five years prior, she had felt sad, lonely, and unlovable. She loved being in a close relationship, so the divorce had really thrown her off emotionally. She told me, "No one would ever want an 'older' woman with eight children!" So we did the Work on that thought, and she responded to my four questions:

1. Is it true that no one would ever want a forty-eight-year-old woman with eight children? "Yes," she said, "No one wants that baggage."

2. Can you *absolutely* know that it is true that no one would ever want a forty-eight-year-old woman with eight children? "No," she said, "Of course, I can't know that for sure."

3. How do you feel when you think this particular thought? "I feel sad, hopeless, and very lonely."

4. Who would you be or how would you feel if you didn't have this particular thought? "I would feel much happier, more optimistic, and probably look more available."

Turnaround—"No one would ever want a forty-eight-year-old woman with eight children." What is the opposite? "Someone will want me and my family." Okay . . . which is truer? "I suppose I don't know," she said, "but if I act like no one will want me, then no one will want me." After cleaning her thoughts and getting on the program to unleash the power of her brain, Celeste started dating again.

To her amazement, she had no problem finding nice men to date who were happy to spend time in a big family. Two years later when I received Celeste's wedding invitation in the mail, there was a personal note that read, "No, it's not true!"

All of us need a way to correct our thoughts. Just think about what happens to all the women like Celeste who let the ANTs dominate their lives, whether in their relationships or at work or with their money. I have seen these four questions dramatically change people's lives and I know they can do the same for you.

Aniko Kills Her ANTs

When Aniko came to our clinic, she was just dragging through the day. An information technology specialist in her early thirties, she had been through a painful breakup with her boyfriend about six months before. Aniko had been more serious about this man than she had about any previous partner, and she had even been hoping to settle down and start a family with him, so when he left, it hit her really hard. She found herself bursting into tears at odd moments, especially the week before her period. On the weekends, she was often so exhausted that she spent one or both days in bed. She had also gained 15 pounds, which made her feel even worse. "I should be able to shake this off," she told me. "But I just can't."

Aniko's SPECT scan confirmed that she had excessive activity in her anxiety centers, causing her to predict the worst. I gave her a regimen of a brain-healthy diet and started her on an exercise program, which I knew would help with her mood, her energy levels, and her weight.

Aniko also needed to soothe her emotions and discipline her mind. I worked with Aniko to identify the ANTs that plagued her the most, which in her case were "always" thinking ("No one will ever love me"), thinking with feelings ("I feel all alone; therefore I *am* all alone"), and fortune-telling ("I'll never have a baby or a family of my own").

Working with Aniko, I found she really gravitated to the four questions. So when Aniko told herself, "No one will ever love me," I asked her to kill the ANT by using Katie's technique. Here's how it worked:

> ANIKO: No one will ever love me!
>
> QUESTION 1: Is that true?
>
> ANIKO: Yes, I just said so! No one will ever love me!
>
> QUESTION 2: Can you absolutely know it's true?
>
> ANIKO: Well, no, I guess not *absolutely*. I guess it *might* not be true . . .
>
> QUESTION 3: What happens when you believe that thought?
>
> ANIKO: I feel sad, lonely, miserable, discouraged . . .
>
> QUESTION 4: Who would you be without that thought?
>
> ANIKO: I might feel more confident. I might be a person who could someday find love.

Turnaround—Someone will love me.

Questioning her negative thoughts helped Aniko to understand that they were only thoughts, not reality. She also used another powerful ANT-killing technique that I teach: identifying the ANT and reframing it into a more accurate statement. Here is how Aniko worked with her ANT "I feel all alone; therefore I *am* all alone."

> ANT: I feel all alone; therefore I *am* all alone.
>
> TYPE OF ANT: Thinking with my feelings
>
> REFRAMING: Even though I *feel* alone, there are a lot of people who care about me—my sister, my best friend, my favorite

cousin, my parents. These people would be there if I asked them for help or even just for a hug. I do miss my boyfriend. But I guess I am only alone if I decide to be.

Killing the ANTs helped Aniko soothe her brain. Although sometimes she still felt sad about not being in a relationship, she generally felt much happier, calmer, and more optimistic. As a result, when a new co-worker asked her out, Aniko was able to imagine good possibilities for the relationship and to go on the date in a cheerful, positive frame of mind. "Even if this relationship doesn't work out," she told me, "I would never even have given it a chance the way I was acting before. Being that negative meant I was never going to find anybody! Now . . . we'll see."

Byron Katie's brain provides the most powerful evidence of this technique. As I wrote above, before she found the ability to question her mind she suffered for many years. But the four questions gave her peace. I met Katie in 2005 and we immediately became close friends. She worked with people I loved to help them discipline their minds and I worked with people she loved to help balance their brains. Over time, I scanned Katie's brain. It looked like that of a person who suffers greatly. Yet Katie was at peace. It was clear evidence to me that doing the Work can help override significant brain problems.

Vulnerability to ANT Infestations

You may find that you're especially prey to your ANTs the week before your period or during the hormonally challenging times of perimenopause and menopause. Your brain-healthy habits are especially critical during those times! Try not to seek the easy answer by reaching for a sweet food or a drink or by popping a pill. Instead, discipline your mind by killing the ANTs and using the Four Questions. Make these exercises part of your life to have a disciplined mind.

And while you're at it, to really solidify them in your head, teach them to your friends, children, co-workers—anyone who will listen. Teaching others allows them to be anchored in your own mind.

View "The Four Questions"

Hypnosis and Meditation: Turn on Your Brain to Turn It Off

Hypnosis and meditation are both powerful ways to soothe your mind and help you create a state of deep relaxation. I have used them in my practice for over three decades and know they are fast and easy ways to calm the mind. Interestingly, both of these "seemingly deep relaxation" techniques actually stimulate or turn on the brain. Studies from Belgium and Canada have shown that hypnosis increases blood flow and activity in the attention areas of the brain and the left hemisphere. It also decreases the perception of pain in the areas of the brain that perceive pain. In our studies, and those done by others, meditation also boosts blood flow to the brain, especially to the PFC, the most human, thoughtful part of the brain.

The neuroscience research on both of these techniques fooled me. Since I have seen myself and my patients obtain deep levels of relaxation using hypnosis and meditation, I thought they would be calming to the brain and we would ultimately see lower overall activity. Yet the opposite proved true. It seems that you have to turn your brain on in order to turn it off. These findings make sense when you consider that the PFC serves an inhibitory function and acts like the brain's brake.

Hypnosis—The PFC helps to calm the more primitive, emotional brain centers (the limbic system), which have been described by our psychiatrist in Reston, Virginia, Joe Annabali, "as being like a bunch of wild horses—you really can't totally control wild horses, but if you can get a hand on their reins, you might be able to influence which direction the horses are running."

Tana often uses my sleep hypnosis audio to slip into a peaceful slumber. She tells me, "I can't listen to the hypnosis audio and the chatter inside my head at the same time." During stressful times, she says, "If I still hear the chatter, I just turn up the volume."

You can listen to my hypnosis audios for anxiety, sleep, pain, weight loss, and peak performance online at www.amensolution.com.

Access audios in the "Relaxation Room/Hypnosis"

Alternatively, here are instructions on how to put yourself into a simple hypnotic trance to boost your brain and soothe your mind. Do not try to do this while driving or operating heavy machinery.

- Focus your eyes on a spot and count slowly to twenty. Let your eyes feel heavy as you count and close them before or as you get to twenty.
- Take four very slow, deep breaths, and as you do feel your belly and chest rise and fall with each breath in and out.
- Progressively tighten and relax the muscles in your feet, legs, arms and then hands.
- Imagine yourself walking down a staircase while you count backward from ten (this will give you the feeling of "going down" or becoming relaxed).
- Using of all of your senses, imagine going to a beautiful place you associate with relaxation, such as a lake, beach, or mountain.

- After spending ten to fifteen minutes in your special place, allow yourself to come back to full consciousness. If you fall asleep, it means that likely you are not getting enough sleep.

I still use this technique when I am stressed, and recently, I had the opportunity to use it to help my daughter.

On the Fourth of July we had a party at our house. As the fireworks started outside, our eight-year-old daughter Chloe was creating her own fireworks in our kitchen. My wife had created a new dessert for the party, a combination of coconut and almond butter. Chloe decided to heat it up, at her mom's direction. But when she took it out of the microwave she tested it with her finger. That is when the screaming started. It was too hot and the concoction stuck to her finger. She tried to shake it off, wiped it off with a towel, and then stuck her finger in her mouth. Then she put her hand in ice water, aloe gel, and then ice cubes. Her pain and frustration escalated as she unraveled and the ANTs started to take over. "I'm so stupid," she said. "Why did I do that?" She was having trouble calming herself down. Her mother gave her ibuprofen for the pain and started putting her to bed. But Chloe was not calming down.

The ANTs were now coming in droves. "I can't do this. It's too much. I can't take it. I'm so stupid. I can't believe I did it. I wish I could go back and do it over."

Tana tried to distract her by reading to her, but it didn't work. She then prayed with her, but Chloe couldn't focus. Nothing worked, so Tana walked into my office and said I needed to help.

I sat on Chloe's bed and assessed the situation. Like I had done for many patients in the hospital, I used a simple hypnotic trance to calm her. Using the outline above, I had her focus on a spot on the wall, close her eyes, and start to relax her body and slow her breathing. I then asked her to imagine walking down a flight of stairs as I counted backward from ten. Then I had her imagine going to a special park that she imagined with all of her senses, where it was safe and she was with her mother and friends. Then I had her imagine going into a warm pool. The water had special healing powers that soothed and helped her finger, taking away the pain. The water helped to calm her thoughts and her body. She did not need to be so hard on herself. We all make mistakes. Being angry only made the pain worse.

Visibly, Chloe was much more relaxed and started to drift off to sleep. The park and special healing pool was a place she could go back to anytime she was upset or needed to calm down. Then Chloe fell asleep. Quietly, we left her room, wondering how she would do. But we did not see her until the next morning, and even though she had a blister on her finger, she said it didn't hurt, and all was well. "Everyone makes mistakes," she said. "I guess that was one of mine."

This technique is very powerful with children and with adults too.

Meditation—Decades of research have shown that meditation and prayer calm stress and enhance brain function. At the Amen Clinics, we performed a SPECT study, sponsored by the Alzheimer's Research and Prevention Foundation, on a Kundalini yoga form of meditation called Kirtan Kriya. We scanned people on one day when they were just letting their mind wander and then the next day during a meditation session. For the meditation, the participants recited the following simple sounds known as the five primal sounds: "sa," "ta," "na," and "ma"; the vowel *a* at the end of each sound is drawn out (like "ahhhh") and is considered to be the fifth sound. The meditation involved touching the thumb of each hand to the index finger while chanting "sa," the middle finger while chanting "ta," the ring finger while chanting "na," and the pinkie finger while chanting "ma." The sounds and fingering were repeated for two minutes whispering, four minutes silently, two minutes whispering, and two minutes out loud.

Kirtan Kriya Fingertip Movements

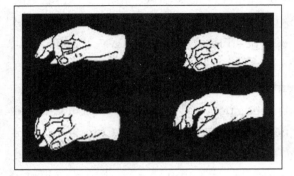

The SPECT scans taken after the meditation showed decreases in activity in the left parietal lobes, which some believe indicates a decreased awareness of time and space. They also showed significant increases in activity in the PFC, which showed in our group that meditation helped to tune people in, not out. We also observed increased activity in the right temporal lobe, an area that has been associated with spirituality.

Will, age forty-five, one of our Kirtan Kriya research subjects, got lost on his way to the clinic and was forty-five minutes late to his appointment. His SPECT scan showed severe damage to the left front side of his brain. When I asked him about it, he told me that at age twenty-one, he'd had a severe motorcycle accident. It was after the accident that he started meditating. This finding on SPECT is often associated with depression and irritability. Yet he was happy and peaceful, if directionally challenged. His story reminds me of Byron Katie's, where using mind discipline techniques can significantly help to soothe brain troubles.

My friend Andy Newberg at Thomas Jefferson University has also used brain SPECT imaging to study the neurobiology of meditation, in part because it is a spiritual state easily duplicated in the laboratory. He scanned nine Buddhist monks before and during prolonged meditation. The scan revealed distinctive changes in brain activity as the mind went into a meditative state. Specifically, activity decreased in the parts of the brain involved in generating a sense of three-dimensional orientation in space. Losing one's sense of physical place could account for the spiritual feeling of transcendence, being beyond space and time, being everywhere and nowhere and united with God and the universe. They also found increased activity in the PFC, associated with attention span and thoughtfulness. Meditation seemed to tune people in, not out. Another functional brain imaging study of transcendental meditation showed calming in the anterior cingulate and basal ganglia, diminishing anxiety and worries and fostering relaxation.

The benefits of meditation go far beyond soothing your mind. Studies have shown that it also improves attention and planning, reduces depression and anxiety, decreases sleepiness, and protects the brain from cognitive decline associated with normal aging. In a study from researchers at UCLA, the hippocampus and frontal cortex were found to be significantly larger in people who meditate regularly. Meditation has also been found to aid in weight loss, reduce muscle tension, and tighten the skin.

A lot of people think it takes years of practice to learn how to meditate. It doesn't. A fascinating Chinese study done by the neuroscientist (and my friend) Dr. Yiyuan Tang showed that people who received just twenty minutes of daily meditation training for five days showed a significant decrease in stress-related cortisol. You don't need to devote big chunks of time to the practice of meditation. In my clinical practice, I often recommend meditation as an integral part of a treatment plan. Many of my patients have reported back that they feel calmer and less stressed after just a few minutes of daily meditation.

If the whole concept of meditation seems a little too New Age-y for you, take note that you can do it just about anywhere, anytime. You don't have to sit cross-legged on the floor or burn incense or any of those things you might associate with meditation. If you are at work, you can simply close the door to your office, sit in your chair, close your eyes, and relax for a few moments by taking five to ten slow, deep breaths. At home, you can sit on the edge of your bed after you wake up and spend a couple of minutes calming your mind by taking slow, deep breaths and imagining yourself in the most beautiful places in the world.

I give my patients the five-five-five rule. Breathe in slowly for five seconds, hold your breath for five seconds, and then slowly breathe out, taking five seconds. Repeat this five to ten times.

You can do a twelve-minute meditation along with me online in the "Relaxation Room" at www.amensolution.com.

 Access a twelve-minute meditation in the "Relaxation Room"

Other mind-soothing and mind-discipline games and techniques found in our online community include:

MyCalmBeat
e-Catch the Feeling
Positive Reflections
e-Self Regulate
Affirm
Thought Challenger
e-Motion Well-being
e-Positive Spin
e-Motion Happy

SOCIAL CONNECTIONS

In soothing your mind, it is critical never to underestimate the power of being around the right people. Start to observe the moods and attitudes of those around you. Do your best to keep angry, irritable people and their moods and mind-sets from rubbing off on you.

My sister Mary lost her husband to cancer, and then fifteen years later she lost her fiancé to a sudden cardiac arrest. Yet Mary was able to stay strong, in large part because she had a supportive family and many, many friends who reached out to her and nurtured her in her time of need. It was not an accident that Mary had so many supportive people in her life. For decades, Mary had nurtured her relationships with her family and friends, and when she needed them most, they were there. If you are feeling down and being infested by the ANTs, or you have monkey-mind thoughts running wildly through your mind, this is when you should get busy spending time with your support group. If you do not have a support group, then consider developing your own at church, in your neighborhood, or by volunteering for a worthy cause.

SPIRITUAL HEALTH

Having a deep sense of meaning and purpose helps to keep you happy and motivated and goes a long way to staving off the thoughts that try to steal your happiness.

Stacie Mathewson suffered greatly when her son struggled with severe drug abuse. After he had a serious overdose and almost died, Stacie decided she had to do something about it. She started a sober college program at the University of Nevada in Reno and a similar program at a local community college. Then she started working on developing drug prevention programs in high schools. Others took notice of her work and asked her to be on the board of directors at the Betty Ford Center. Through Stacie's efforts, she was able to get an amendment to a California law that courts considering child custody to take into account either parent's continual or habitual use of prescribed controlled substances. We worked together on creating brain-healthy treatment programs. Stacie's work gave her a deep sense of meaning and purpose, which helped to corral her ANTs and diminish her own suffering, as well as the suffering of countless others.

To Medicate or Not Medicate?

I am a classically trained psychiatrist and have prescribed medications for a long time. I am not opposed to using medicine for emotional or behavioral problems. I am just opposed to their indiscriminant use. Given the expense and side effects of medications for anxiety and depression, I prefer to first try natural treatments such as exercise, meditation, ANT therapy, and natural supplements targeted toward a patient's particular brain type. If medication is needed, be cautious and proceed slowly. Use our brain-typing method above as a guide to help you determine the type of medication best suited to you. Always consult with your health care provider.

Hour 6 Exercise—Get ANT Therapy and Answer the Work's Four Questions

1. GET ANT THERAPY

1. Whenever you feel sad, mad, nervous, or out of control, draw two lines vertically down a piece of paper, dividing it into three columns.
2. In the first column, write down the ANTs going through your brain.
3. In the second column, identify the type of ANT or negative thought. Therapists typically describe nine different types of ANTs.

4. In the third column, talk back, correct, and eradicate the ANTs. If you were like me, you were good at talking back to your parents when you were a teenager, In the same way, you need to learn to be good at talking back to the lies you tell yourself.

2. ANSWER THE WORK'S FOUR QUESTIONS

Write down disturbing thoughts that upset you. Then ask yourself.

1. Is it true?
2. Can you absolutely know that it's true?
3. How do you react when you believe that thought?
4. Who would you be without the thought? Or, how would you feel if you didn't have the thought?

Turnaround—After you answer the four questions, you then take the original thought and completely turn it around to its opposite, and ask yourself whether the opposite of the original thought that is causing your suffering is not true or even truer than the original thought. Then, take the turned-around thought and apply it to yourself and to the other person, if someone else is involved in the thought.

7

GET CONTROL OF THE FEMALE BRAIN

CONQUER CRAVINGS, WEIGHT ISSUES, AND ADDICTIONS

Boosting self-control is the seventh step to unleash the power of the female brain.
The human race is challenged more than ever before to demonstrate our mastery, not over nature but of ourselves.

—RACHEL CARSON

Teri came up to me after a lecture. She was part of the Daniel Plan, our cooperative program with Saddleback Church.

"Before I met you," she said, "I knew I was fat and I knew I was not attractive, but I always thought I had a great mind. Then I listened to you talk about the 'dinosaur syndrome'—as your weight goes up, the size and function of your brain goes down. That totally did me in. Last year, my father died of Alzheimer's disease and I want no part of it. That was when I really got serious about my health. In the last eight months I have lost 90 pounds and feel better than ever. Thank you!"

The dinosaur syndrome that Teri referred to is a term I coined as a stark reminder of the importance of keeping your weight under control.

Teri's Transformed Brain and Body

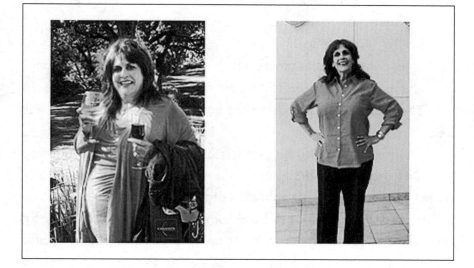

There are eighteen studies that report an inverse correlation between weight increase and brain size and function decrease. Cyrus Raji and his team at the University of Pittsburgh published the first study and it caused me to lose 20 pounds. I am not going to do anything purposefully that damages my brain.

A few weeks after reading Dr. Raji's study, I was in Pittsburgh for a meeting at a large health care company, where we were considering a joint project. The marketing director, Tom, was morbidly obese, which upset me. If you don't live the message of your organization, then you are not a good messenger, which is one reason why overweight physicians have trouble helping their patients get well through lifestyle interventions. As part of the visit, Tom took me to dinner at a local restaurant. When I heard him order two soufflés for dessert, I just couldn't stand it anymore and told him that he wanted to avoid the dinosaur syndrome.

Tom laughed and said, "What's the dinosaur syndrome?"

"Don't you know that there are studies now that say as your weight goes up, the actual physical size and function of your brain go down? The first study was done in this very town."

"Really?" Tom replied.

"Tom, do you want to progress in your career, or are you finished?"

"I have a lot of work left to do. I am not anywhere near done."

"Then you need to have a healthy brain and get serious about your weight."

A month later, Tom wrote an email to me that he had lost 17 pounds. He didn't want to be a dinosaur. It was after receiving that email I decided I had to start talking about the dinosaur syndrome. I never want to hurt anyone's feelings, but I feel compelled to tell the truth. Being overweight or obese has a significant negative impact on brain health. Learning about the dinosaur syndrome worked for Teri and Tom and countless others who have written to me.

One of the greatest joys in my life has been helping people get control over their brains and lives. Like Teri and Tom, you can make your brain better, even if you have been bad to it. We have proven this in our clinical practice again and again at the Amen Clinics.

Here are six very clear steps to gain control over your mind, your weight, and any addictions you may suffer:

1. Develop brain envy, and know why you care. Do you have anchor images to remind yourself every day why you must do the right things for your brain?

2. Get a comprehensive evaluation in which you learn your important numbers and your brain type. This step will allow you to target the help specifically to *your* brain. One-size-fits-all approaches don't work.

3. Get very serious about avoiding anything that hurts your

brain. You cannot be in control of your mind when your brain is in a toxic, traumatic, or malnourished environment.

4. Engage in regular brain-healthy habits to boost your brain's reserve and engage all of its healing processes.

5. Boost the quality of your decisions to gain more control over your life.

6. Learn and implement the science of change.

None of these strategies are hard. They just take a little forethought and need to be applied consistently over time. This book has already covered the first four steps in detail. In this chapter, I will cover steps 5 and 6. But first, take a moment to read about Arianna. Her story highlights the importance of avoiding anything that hurts your brain.

Arianna, twenty-three, struggled with bulimia. She hated herself whenever she gave in to the temptation to make herself throw up. After her evaluation and treatment plan, she did much better, but after about four months of treatment, she relapsed. When I asked her to describe in detail what happened, she said, "I went with friends to a restaurant where we shared a bottle of wine. I had about two glasses. Even though I promised myself I wouldn't eat because I'd already had dinner, after the wine I ordered a plate of nachos. Then, about midnight I really hated myself, so I purged."

As Arianna and I discussed the situation, it dawned on her that the problem would never have happened if she hadn't drunk the wine. It was the alcohol that lowered her impulse control, which led to the nachos, self-loathing, vomiting, and more self-loathing. When you avoid the things that hurt your brain, the quality of your decisions is much better. After that relapse, Arianna stopped both her drinking and her purging behaviors. Of course, bulimia is more complex, but it is often related to alcohol, poor sleep, poor nutrition, or low blood sugar states, which lead to troubled behavior.

BOOST THE QUALITY OF YOUR DECISIONS

The best way to reduce stress in your life is to stop screwing up.

—Roy Baumeister, Ph.D.

Many people face a number of obstacles that jeopardize high-quality decisions. These barriers can include food pushers, energy zappers, and financial concerns. Consistently making great decisions is not hard if you put your brain in a position to help you make them. In order to boost the quality of your decisions, here are the most important steps:

- Start with clear focus. Know your goals and look at them every day.
- Make decisions about your health ahead of time. It is good to have a few simple rules, such as no bread or drinking alcohol at restaurants before meals, as they both lower PFC function and have a negative impact on decisions.
- Make sure to eat breakfast, and include some high-quality protein to balance your blood sugar levels. Low blood sugar levels are associated with lower overall blood flow to the brain and more bad decisions. Make sure to eat throughout the day to maintain your blood sugar levels.
- Eliminate sugar and artificial sweeteners. These often trigger cravings and poor decisions.
- Get at least seven hours of sleep at night. Less than that is associated with lower blood flow to the brain and more bad decisions.
- Don't put yourself in vulnerable situations. Think ahead. If you know you are going to a party that is likely to serve unhealthy food, eat before you go so you won't feel hungry and lose control. My wife often brings food with her to gatherings, just to have something in case of emergency low blood sugar.

Many people face a number of obstacles that jeopardize high quality decisions, such as food pushers, energy zappers, and financial concerns. When you start living a brain-healthy life, it can make those around you uncomfortable, especially if they have a lot of their own bad brain habits. Deep down, some people, even those who love you the most, don't want you to succeed because it will make them feel like more of a failure. For others, their habits are so ingrained that they simply don't know how to react to your new lifestyle. Many of my patients notice this kind of behavior with their families, friends, and co-workers. This is why it is so important for you to take control of your life. You need to be prepared for the obstacles that will come your way so you can deal with them and continue to make good decisions.

You will be better prepared to handle challenges if you live by the acronym HALT, which is a common term used in addiction treatment programs. HALT stands for:

- Don't get too *h*ungry. Eat frequent, small, high-quality meals and take nutritional supplements to optimize your brain and balance your blood sugar.
- Don't get too *a*ngry. Maintain control over your emotions and don't let negative thinking patterns rule your life. See Chapter 6 to kill the ANTs.
- Don't get too *l*onely. Social skills and a positive social network are critical to maintaining freedom from the bad habits that control you. Enlist a team of supporters and healthy role models.
- Don't get too *t*ired. Make sleep a priority to boost brain function and improve judgment and self-control.

Many people, companies, and our society will try to push things on you that threaten your brain health and trigger old destructive habits. As a society, we're bombarded with messages about food, coffee, cigarettes, alcohol, shopping, and more. TV commercials, billboards, and radio ads are constantly showing us images of happy, attractive people enjoying greasy fast food, judgment-impairing cocktails, and dehydrating caffeinated drinks, all of which reduce brain function and self-control. Movies depict gorgeous celebrities smoking, drinking, fighting, and engaging in reckless behaviors, which can fire up those emotional memory centers in the brain and trigger a return to old habits.

Corporations are highly skilled at pushing us to eat and drink things that are not good for our brain health. Restaurants and fast-food places train employees to "upsell" as a way to increase sales and, subsequently, expand our waistlines. Here are some of the sneaky tactics food sellers use to try to get you to eat and drink more:

> "Do you want to supersize that for only thirty-nine cents?"
> "Do you want fries with your meal?"
> "Do you want bread first?" (This makes you hungrier so you eat more!)
> "Do you want an appetizer?"
> "Do you want another drink?" (This decreases your judgment.)
> "Do you want a larger drink? It is a better deal!"

"No!" is the brain-smart answer to all of these questions. Eating or drinking more than you need just because it's more economical will cost you far more in the long run.

Unfortunately, spouses, friends, co-workers, neighbors, and even children can also make it very difficult for you to stay on track regardless of the type of behaviors you are trying to conquer. A friend who smokes may light up in front of you even though you are trying to quit. A neighbor might show up with a box of home-baked brownies for your birthday when you are trying to curb your sugar intake. At work, your supervisor may invite your team to go to happy hour for drinks, or someone in the operations department may offer you candy from the bowl on her desk.

Recently, I came home to a houseful of girls. Chloe had just finished third grade and she invited friends over to swim. As I walked into the house, a mother of one of her friends walked into the house with a box full of greasy French fries, cheeseburgers, and large sodas. I thought to myself, "This is going to be interesting."

The woman offered them to my wife with a look of pride. "I was at a party and they had food, so I brought you some."

Tana politely said, "That is not the type of food we eat."

"Oh, come on, it's fries, cheeseburgers, and sodas. Everyone likes them."

"Not everyone," Tana said, still trying to maintain a friendly tone.

The woman looked at me, "Don't you eat this way?"

"I don't think I've seen this kind of food in our home for years. Thanks for thinking of us, but you can take it with you," I said, trying less hard than Tana to be polite.

"I'll just leave it in case you get hungry." And with that she left with her daughter.

I looked at Tana and she looked at me. "What just happened," I said, "It was like we just had a food-pusher invasion." I took the food and promptly threw it out. I didn't want to start craving after something that would hurt me.

People aren't the only pushers. Places and environmental cues can trigger problem behaviors. Almost everywhere you go, you will see reminders that tempt you to engage in your old unhealthy behaviors. In the addiction field, they are called slippery places. Go to the movies and you'll have to drive by the fast-food place where you used to hang out with your friends and get high. Take a cruise to Alaska because you want to see the beautiful scenery and you'll have to face unbelievably copious amounts of food and desserts at the buffet and free-flowing alcohol. Join your colleagues at a convention in Las Vegas and you'll have to deal with all sorts of temptations that threaten your brain health and recovery.

Learning to deal with and say no to all of these pushers in the home, on the town, at work, and at school is critical to your success.

Ten More Tips for Making Great Decisions

1. If you are going to a dinner with friends or family, call ahead to inform the host that you are on a special brain-healthy diet and won't be able to eat certain foods.

2. When invited to parties where people may be smoking, drinking, or doing drugs, either don't go or go with a friend who supports you in your efforts and will take you home if you feel tempted.

3. Be upfront with food pushers. Explain that you are trying to eat a more balanced diet and that when they offer you cake, chips, or pizza, it makes it more difficult for you.

4. Instead of going out for a smoke break or drinks with friends, choose activities that aren't centered on your unwanted behavior, such as going for a walk.

5. When people offer seconds, tell them you are pleasantly full. If they insist, explain that you are trying to watch your calories. If they continue to push extra helpings on you, ask them why they are bent on sabotaging your efforts to be healthy.

6. I know some people who will accept a piece of cake or a cocktail and then toss it in the trash or the sink as soon as the host turns away. It is better to be wasteful on occasion than to endanger your recovery.

7. Avoid people who are negative, gossipy, or complainers. They bring you down.

8. Tell your host you don't drink alcohol, period.

9. Take a healthy sack lunch so you don't have to eat from the cafeteria at work or school.

10. Commit to taking control of your own body and don't let other people make you fat and stupid.

LEARN AND IMPLEMENT THE SCIENCE OF CHANGE

Scientists have studied how the brain can facilitate change, whether it is to lose weight, beat an addiction, or change personal habits. Here are seven steps.

1. You Have to Decide What You Truly Want—This will help your PFC to lead the way. Your brain makes happen what it sees. Define the goal.

Create a vivid and believable "future of success" in great detail. Ask yourself how you'll feel in one, five, and ten years if you stay the course and succeed. The answer? Amazing, healthy, energetic, cognitively better than you have ever been (wisdom plus mental energy).

Create a vivid and believable "future of failure" in great detail. Ask yourself how you'll feel in one, five, and ten years if you *don't* stop your negative behaviors. What will your life look like going forward? A smaller brain, early disease, and earlier death.

2. Know Your Critical Behaviors—Ask yourself what you need to get healthy. For any problem, such as overweight or an addiction, it is critical to know the important behaviors you need to do to reach your goal; then practice them over and over. Examples include:

- Get your blood work done, so you do not miss something important, such as low vitamin D, thyroid, or testosterone levels.
- Know your brain type (impulsive, compulsive, sad, or anxious), and get help for it.
- Get plenty of sleep—this is so important to maintain healthy PFC function.

- Balance your blood sugar to kill the cravings.
- Consistently eat whole, high-quality food but not too much.
- Journal your calories, so you do not overspend.
- Eliminate any foods you may have allergies to, such as milk or wheat products.
- Avoid the places that trigger cravings.
- Control your thoughts, so you don't have to medicate them with food or drugs.
- Get consistent exercise.
- Take proper nutritional supplementation.
- Rely on group support.

3. Identify Your Most Vulnerable Moments—Be curious about your behavior. Investigating your slipups and bad days can be so instructive if you take the time to really think about them.

Martha, fifty-three, a highly successful attorney, came into my office feeling sad and ashamed. I initially saw her for panic attacks and drinking excessive amounts of alcohol. After a few months, she had made great progress and had completely stopped drinking. But then she slipped and went on a weekend binge after she had a major fight with her husband.

"I'll never beat this," she told me. Then she stopped herself and said, "I know that is not true." We had worked on the four questions over and over. "I just get so frustrated when I fail."

I went to the whiteboard in my office and drew for her this graph on how people change.

"When people come to see me," I told her, "they have good days and bad days, but usually their days are not very good. Then we work together to change things and they get better. But it is never that they just get better and stay there. There is an up-and-down course. Over time, they feel much better and usually stay that way. But it is the down times, the slipups, and the setbacks that teach us most of what we need

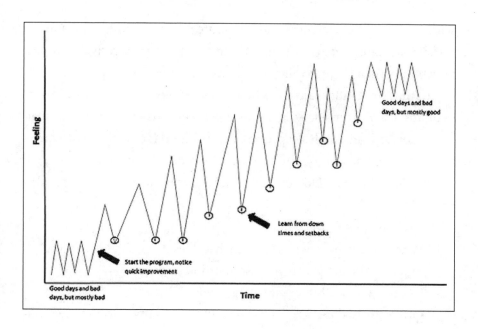

to know if we embrace them and take time to learn from them. We have to turn bad days into useful information."

Former White House chief of staff Rahm Emanuel once said that you never want a serious crisis to go to waste. Slipups and setbacks are the same way. Study them, learn from them, be curious. In my experience, the most successful people embrace their mistakes to learn from them.

So Martha and I investigated her relapse from a brain science perspective. The week before her relapse she had stayed up late every night working on a difficult case. On three of the nights she got fewer than five hours of sleep. In addition, she became erratic in her eating habits, and she did not take time to work out. She skipped her supplements and also started eating fast food, including gluten, which she knew she was sensitive to. An inappropriate amount of sleep, erratic eating habits, and a lack of exercise all contributed to lower activity and blood flow to her brain. When those factors combined with a difficult interaction with her husband, who also had a stressful week, she became overwhelmed with a sense of hopelessness and had more ANTs starting to invade her mind. Ultimately, she got drunk to shut up the noisy negative thoughts, which only then increased her self-loathing—and the relapse was on.

Rather than judge herself as bad, I encouraged her to be a good student and learn from the episode, as it was very instructive. She needed to be more diligent with sleep, exercise, and good food, along with questioning her negative thoughts that easily got out of control.

I asked Martha, "Do you have a GPS system in your car that talks to you?"

"Yes," she replied.

"When you make a wrong turn, what does he or she say to you?"

"Make the next legal turn, or something like that."

"Does it start yelling or swearing at you?"

With a smile she said, "They wouldn't sell many of those GPS systems. Of course not."

"But isn't this what you are doing to yourself when you make a mistake? Whenever you make a mistake, learn from it, turn around, and go in a better direction."

Be the investigator and the subject!

Change is a process that occurs in steps. If you pay attention, the bad times can be more instructive than the good times. Journaling is key to helping keep track of the good times and the bad times. Know when are you most vulnerable (e.g., when you haven't slept, have forgotten to eat breakfast, allowed too much time to pass between meals or while at parties or social gatherings).

Create simple rules for vulnerable times, such as:

1. I'll eat healthy foods before bad ones.
2. I'll split my orders.
3. I'll eat veggies first.

4. I'll eat something before I go to the ball game to avoid being tempted by the caramel apples.

5. I'll use smaller plates.

6. I'll allow myself to cheat on my diet—but only after reading my motivation list and calling supportive friends. (This rule introduces a delay and social support.)

7. I'll be aware of the impulse and then focus on something else, like taking a walk, repeating a poem, or drinking a glass of water, until the impulse goes away.

In Kerry Patterson and colleagues' book, *Change Anything: The New Science of Personal Success*, there is a phrase to sum up these steps: "Turn bad days into good data."

4. Learn to Love What You Hate—If you are ever going to succeed at changing, you have to disarm your impulses and make the right choices pleasurable. Learn how to find what you love about not being inebriated, or identify great low-calorie, highly nutritious foods. Learn to find what you love about exercise. One of my friends told me she hated exercise, but she loved walking with her children. Mind-set is key.

The only way you can sustain change is to change what brings you pleasure!

Connect to who you are becoming . . . think like a healthy person. How would a healthy person order this meal or act in this vulnerable situation? Willpower is a skill; if you can distract yourself for just a minute, temptations often go away.

Be careful about giving in to your own bad behavior. You may be causing your own behavior disorder. I was once with a patient who was struggling with her weight. She said she often felt as though she *had* to give in to her cravings. She had two teenage daughters, one of whom had tantrums whenever she did not get her way. "And if you were to give into your daughter's temper tantrums," I prompted her, "would she get better or worse?" "Worse, of course," my patient said. When you give in to your own tantrums. you are creating your own internal behavior disorder, which is ruining your health and killing you early. Be a loving, effective parent to yourself.

5. Who You Spend Time with Matters!—Turn accomplices into friends. Cultivating bad habits—and good ones—is a team sport. Habits need lots of accomplices to start and sustain them. Friends, mentors, or coaches are people who support your positive behaviors. Ask for their help. Adding friends improves your chances for success up to 40 percent, and this is especially true for weight loss and fitness.

The nutritional gatekeeper of the family *must* become your friend and supporter in order for you to be successful. This is why it is important to *stop* spending money on food
that hurts your family, employees, or friends. It leaves them vulnerable to failure, it hurts their chances for success, and it is a matter of your own integrity.

Accomplices are people who encourage or are complicit with your negative behaviors. If you want to change your behavior, you need to change your friends or turn accomplices into friends or people with whom you spend little or no time.

Many accomplices can change into friends if you have crucial conversations with them. Explain what these people can start doing to help you, and what they can stop doing, and what they can continue doing.

6. Make Your Space Work for You—Most people are blinded by the myriad ways our environment controls us. Our surroundings powerfully control what we think, how we feel, and how we

act. If you want to take control of your own life, you have to take
control of your surroundings.

Build fences that keep good things in and bad things out:

- Clean out the kitchen.
- Put a fruit bowl on the table.
- Shop the outside edges of the grocery store, where the fresh
  foods are, and avoid the internal aisles as much as possible,
  because that is where the packaged foods are.
- Put a mental fence across the middle of most restaurant
  menus where the high-calorie appetizers and alcoholic drinks
  are.
- Eliminate the alcohol or drugs in the house.

Manage distance:

- Place exercise equipment closer.
- Place bad food far away.
- Never go near your trigger places.

Use cues to jolt you out of routine:

- Use personal sayings, such as "Nothing tastes as good as
  healthy feels."
- Put active photos in your office.
- Cues should be placed so that they help you in the crucial
  moments.

Use tools:

- Track your walking with a pedometers.
- Download apps for tracking calories.

- Place a paper calendar in the bathroom to track your weight.
- Use smaller pans, servings bowls and plates to decrease your portions.

7. Stay in the Center of Your Purpose on Earth.—Pray for a blessing on the health of your children, grandchildren, employees, and friends. You are their guide and your guidance will affect them for generations.

THE MISSING LINK

Most of the research and books on change miss a key point. You need a healthy brain to make it happen. If your brain is not right, you're not right. Any successful change requires your physical brain to work in a healthy way. If your brain has been hurt, it is essential to rehabilitate it. Avoiding anything that hurts your brain and engaging in brain-healthy habits is also crucial. Taking care of your physical and brain health is a prerequisite to making and sustaining change.

Hour 7 Exercise—Embrace Your Failures

New neuroscience research reports that there is a significant brain difference between people who learn from their mistakes and those who don't. Using brain scans, it seems that when some people make mistakes, the anxiety centers of their brains become more anxious, causing them to try to avoid thinking about them, whereas for others, the pleasure centers of their brains activate, helping them to embrace their failures and learn from them. If you are going to thrive and improve your behavior to make great decisions and gain better self-control, it is essential to learn from your vulnerable times. For example, for me, I tend to love eating popcorn at movie theaters. But their popcorn is not on my health list. So I have come up with strategies to deal with the popcorn monster, such as eating before going to the movies and bringing in healthy snacks that I do like.

For the next hour, list at least five repetitive mistakes you tend to make. Write about them, why you think they happen repeatedly, and then come up with a list of five strategies to help you overcome the vulnerable times. Here's an example from one of my recent patients:

> MISTAKE: When I go out with friends I often will have two or three glasses of wine. Sometimes that causes me to overeat and I subsequently want to throw up the extra calories. The next day I usually feel awful.
>
> WHY: I developed this habit so I would be accepted when I'm with my friends and feel less anxious, as alcohol helps me relax.

Five Strategies I've planned ahead to Break This Pattern
1. Have a clear goal for the evening before going out (e.g., fun, fellowship, self-control).
2. Order sparkling water with a lime (or the like) and nurse it throughout the evening.
3. Have a healthy meal or snack before we go out to have a healthy blood sugar.
4. Bring healthy snacks with me.
5. Use the ANTs-killing technique or the Work's four questions from chapter 6 if I feel anxious.

8

UNDERSTAND ADD AND THE FEMALE BRAIN

THE HYPERACTIVE "BOYS' CONDITION" THAT RUINS FEMALE LIVES

Overcoming focus issues is the eighth step to
unleash the power of the female brain.
You mean I am not lazy, crazy, or stupid?

—KATE KELLY AND PEGGY RAMUNDO

Check the statements that apply to you:

1. Do you get easily bored?
2. Does your mind frequently wander in conversations?
3. Do you get distracted easily?
4. Do you find yourself often starting conflict?
5. Do you often say things you later regret?
6. Do you often forget to do something you promised?
7. Do you often get distracted during sex?
8. Do you find that your disorganization often causes problems for you?

9. Do you often have anger outbursts with little or no provocation?
10. Does your mind tend to go blank during conversations?
11. Do you need music or the sound of a fan in order to settle your mind before bedtime?

If more than four statements are checked, there is a suspicion for ADD (attention deficit disorder). Reading this chapter may have a profound positive impact on your life.

I met Catherine when she brought her eighteen-year-old son to our clinic. He was having trouble staying on top of his work in college, often missed classes, and didn't turn in assignments, even when he had done them. During our evaluations of children and teenagers at the Amen Clinics, parents fill out our intake questionnaires on themselves. Mental health issues often run in families and we want to make sure that everyone who needs help gets it. Catherine scored very high on the ADD portion of the questionnaire. She decided to make an appointment for herself.

Features of ADD (often referred to as ADHD) have been described since the eighteenth century. Philosopher John Locke described a perplexing group of young students who "try as they might . . . cannot keep their minds from straying." Its hallmark symptoms are short attention span, distractibility, disorganization, restlessness, and impulse control. It is commonly thought of as a disorder of hyperactive, behaviorally troubled boys. Yet it afflicts many girls too, and they are often overlooked, because they tend not to be as hyperactive and have fewer behavior problems. Missing ADD in females, however, can have devastating lifelong effects on their health, mood, relationships, career, and finances.

All of her life Catherine felt stupid. Even though she ended up finishing college, she was labeled as a slow learner in elementary school and junior high school. She felt that she had to try harder than everyone else. Homework took her longer to do than it took her friends. She often didn't go out on weekends because she was overloaded with schoolwork. Even now, she told me, chores around the house took her longer than she (or her husband) thought they should. Catherine struggled with bulimia as a teenager and young woman, and she complained of a long-standing sense of anxiety and restlessness.

She stopped going out to movies. "I can't sit still for more than fifteen minutes at a time. Getting up all the time and walking around irritates others." Because of her distractibility, she would often interrupt her husband in the theatre and ask what just happened or what was said.

She had problems with follow through, often having to pay late fees for her bills even when she had the money.

Her husband complained that Catherine was conflict seeking. "Often I feel like she will just start problems to have a problem," he said. "If we're having a nice day, she'll start to pick at me or bring something up from the past to be upset about. I don't think we have had a whole month in our twenty-five-year marriage without a bad fight."

In addition, Catherine was disorganized. She told me that her closets were a "disaster area." "You have to wear a hard hat when you go in them," was her husband's comment. She was also frequently late.

As part of their evaluations, both Catherine and her son were scanned. They both had a similar SPECT pattern: reasonably healthy brain activity at rest, but poor activity in the PFC with concentration. In my experience, the images of good activity at rest that decrease with concentration perfectly describe people with ADD. The harder they try, the worse it gets for them.

Catherine had a very nice response to treatment. She said her energy was better. She felt more focused and was more effective in her day-to-day life. Her anxiety level settled down and she was able to sit through movies without having to get up or miss part of the plot. Her husband said that she was more relaxed, less negative, and less conflict seeking. Plus, Catherine told me with a smile, "There was a surprise added bonus." I had seen that smile many times before and had a sense of what she would say next. "Because I can focus better, my orgasms are easier and much more intense."

Catherine's ADD Scans (note the deactivation with concentration)

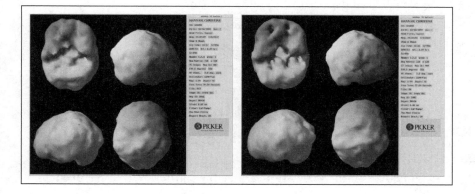

"What do orgasms require?" I often ask audiences in my lectures. Someone will say, "A competent lover." Others may blurt out, "A great imagination." I keep asking until someone says, "Attention." You have to pay attention to the feeling long enough to make it happen. As Catherine's focus improved, her ability to experience ecstasy improved as well.

It is estimated that seventeen million people in the United States have ADD. It is the most common learning and behavioral problem in children and one of the most common problems in adults, leading to job failures, relationship breakups, loneliness, drug abuse, and a tremendous sense of underachievement.

This chapter will explore how ADD affects the female brain, including the myths and misconceptions about ADD, its primary symptoms, different types, and treatments.

Unfortunately, many myths and misconceptions about ADD abound in our society. Here is a list of common falsehoods, as well as the truth, as I see it, about ADD.

The Myths About ADD

- ADD is the flavor of the month illness. It is a fad diagnosis and just an excuse for bad behavior.
- ADD is overdiagnosed. Every child that acts up a bit gets placed on medication.
- ADD is a disorder of hyperactive boys.
- ADD is only a minor problem. We don't need to make such a fuss over it.
- ADD is an American invention, made up by a society seeking simple solutions to complex problems.
- Bad parents or bad teachers cause ADD. If only our society was firmer and stricter with these people there wouldn't be these problems.
- People with ADD should just try harder. We don't need to give them excuses.
- Everyone outgrows ADD by the age of twelve or thirteen.
- Stimulant medication for ADD is dangerous and highly addictive.
- Medication alone is the best treatment for ADD.

The Truth About ADD

- ADD is not new. In 1902, pediatrician George Still described a group of children who were hyperactive, impulsive, and inattentive. Unfortunately, he didn't understand that ADD is a medical disorder, and he labeled these children as "morally defective."
- ADD affects approximately 6 percent of the population, but fewer than 2% receive treatment. Child psychiatrist Peter Jensen found that less than one in eight children who met the diagnostic criteria for ADD were taking medication. Many children, especially girls, with ADD go untreated.

- Many people with ADD are never hyperactive. The nonhyperactive ADD group is often ignored because they do not bring enough negative attention to themselves. They are not a big enough problem. Many of these children, teenagers, or adults are just labeled as willful, lazy, unmotivated, or "not that smart." Females have ADD in high numbers, yet males are diagnosed three to four times more than females. Gender bias issues and the decreased incidence of hyperactivity in females may account for these differences.
- ADD is a serious societal problem.
  - Girls with ADD suffer more than seven times the risk for both antisocial and mood disorders, three times the risk for addictive disorders, and twice the risk for anxiety disorders. They have a higher risk for eating disorders, such as bulimia and obesity.
  - Girls with ADD have more conflicts with their mothers and struggle more in romantic relationships. In one study, 75 percent of people with ADD have interpersonal problems.
  - Teens with ADD are almost three times more likely to drop out of high school (25 percent repeat at least one grade).
  - One study reported that 52 percent of untreated ADD teens and adults abuse drugs or alcohol.
  - People with ADD smoke cigarettes nearly double the general population.
  - People with ADD use medical services three times the general population.
  - There is a higher percentage of motor vehicle accidents, speeding tickets, driving without a license, and suspended or revoked licenses.
  - Parents of ADD children divorce three times more than the general population.

- ADD is found in every country where it has been studied. Our clinics evaluate and treat people from all over the world. We have seen ADD patients from Hong Kong, Lebanon, Ethiopia, West Africa, Israel, and Russia. Having ADD in a nomadic culture often causes the person afflicted to be ostracized from their group, because they have trouble conforming to societal norms.
- Poor parents or teachers certainly can make ADD symptoms worse, but it is not the cause. Genetic features, poor nutrition, and environmental toxins lead the list of causes. The behaviors of these children and adults often make even skilled parents and teachers or spouses appear stressed and inept.
- The harder many people with ADD try, the worse things get. Brain imaging studies show that most people with ADD experience PFC shutdown during concentration tasks. This means that when they try to concentrate, the part of their brain involved with concentration, focus, and follow-through actually shuts down when they need it to turn on. In a sense, their brain betrays them.
- Many people never outgrow ADD and have symptoms that interfere with their whole lives. The statistics say that at least half of those children diagnosed with ADD will have disabling symptoms into adulthood.

As I mentioned above, according to one study, 75 percent of people with untreated ADD have interpersonal problems. Why? In my lectures I often ask the audience the following question: "How many of you are married?" Many in the audience raise their hands. I continue, "Is it helpful for you to say everything you think in your marriage?" The audience laughs. "Of course not," I continue. "Relationships require tact. They require forethought. But when you have low activity in the front part of your brain, as most people with ADD do, you often say the first thing that comes into your mind, which hurts other people's feelings."

The brain is a sneaky organ. We all have weird, crazy, stupid, sexual, violent thoughts that no one should ever hear. It is the front part of our brain that protects us from saying those stupid thoughts out loud. It acts as the brain's brake. I was once at a conference with one of my friends who has ADD and a brain injury. Two obese women were sitting in front of us talking about their weight problem. One woman said to the other, "I don't know why I am so fat. I eat like a bird." My friend looked at me and said loud enough for everyone around us to hear, "Yeah, like a condor." I looked at my friend in total embarrassment. Horrified, my friend put her hand over her mouth and said, "Oh my God, did that thought get out?" I nodded yes as the women moved away from us in disgust.

I agree that many physicians reach for stimulant medications too quickly and that we should try natural treatments first. Yet, when used cautiously, stimulant medications such as Adderall or Ritalin, are generally safe and effective. Ritalin was approved for use in the United States some fifty years ago. We know a great deal about these medications. Work done at Harvard demonstrated that children treated for ADD have a lower risk than non-treated children for drug abuse. In Sweden, researchers report lower arrest records for people with ADD while they are taking their medication. Typically, untreated ADD has more side effects than these medications when they are properly prescribed. But to effectively treat ADD, a comprehensive Four Circles Approach to treatment is essential and must include education, support, exercise, nutrition, dietary supplements, and then, if needed, medication. Unfortunately, medications are the only treatments given to the vast majority of people diagnosed with ADD in America.

Why are there so many myths and negative reactions about ADD when trained physicians know so much about it? The answer is simple. *Until now you couldn't see ADD.* Children, teens, and adults with ADD look like everyone else. Unless you know the story of an ADD person's life, you can't see that he or she has ADD.

Based on our research with tens of thousands of ADD patients using brain SPECT imaging we have been able to see the systems in the brain that are troubled and why it has such a negative impact on behavior. *By actually seeing ADD, the myths fade away and a new era of understanding and effective treatment unfolds.*

HALLMARK SYMPTOMS OF ADD

The hallmark symptoms of ADD are short attention span, distractibility, disorganization, procrastination, and poor internal supervision. Some females are hyperactive, but many are not.

Short attention span is the key symptom of ADD, but it is not short attention span for everything. People with ADD have trouble with regular, routine, everyday attention. The kind of attention that makes life work, such as getting your homework done, paying bills on time, cleaning the house, doing your expense report at work, listening to your spouse, or consistently taking your supplements or medication. For things that are new, novel, highly stimulating, interesting, or frightening, people with ADD can pay attention just fine. It is as though they need stimulation in order to pay attention, which is why they go to scary movies, engage in high-risk activities, and tend to be conflict seeking in their relationships. Many people with ADD play this "Let's Have a Problem" game. If they are upset, they can focus and may even overfocus on the problem. This trait often fools people, even doctors, because if you can pay attention to things you love but not most other things, then people do not think you have ADD; they just think you are lazy.

Distractibility is another common symptom. Most of us can block out things we do not need to think about. Not people with ADD. Their thoughts and conversations tend to bounce around. Their monkey mind is hyperactive. People with ADD also tend to feel everything. They hate garment tags and their clothes have to be just right or they get upset. They are often sensitive to touch and may need white noise at night to sleep otherwise they hear everything in the house. Distractibility often affects a woman's ability to have an orgasm. As mentioned, what does an orgasm require? Attention! You have to pay attention to the feeling long enough to make it happen. After properly treating ADD, many people's sex lives get much better.

Many people with ADD are disorganized. Their rooms, desks, drawers and closets are often a mess. They are also often disorganized about time and tend to be late. You can tell the ADD people at work because they are always ten minutes late and usually show up with a big cup of coffee in their hands. Many people with ADD self-medicate with stimulants, such as caffeine and nicotine.

And many people with ADD have what I call poor internal supervision. They don't think before they say things and they don't think before they do things, which gets them into lots of hot water. Many people with ADD also have trouble with long-term goals. The moment is what matters to them, not five moments from now or ten moments from now but *now.* They wait until the last minute to get things done and have trouble saving for retirement. They also take what I call a crisis management approach to life. It seems as though their life goes from one crisis to the next.

Typical ADD Scans (note the deactivation with concentration)

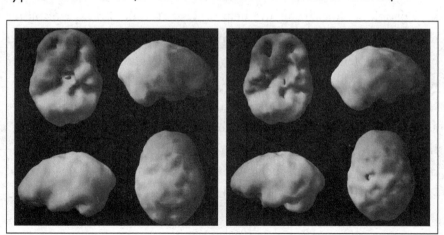

Our research shows that ADD primarily affects the following areas of the brain:

- PFC—the brain's controller of concentration, attention span, judgment, organization, planning, and impulse control
- Anterior cingulate gyrus—the brain's gear shifter
- Temporal lobes—the brain's housing for memory and experience
- Basal ganglia—the area that produces and processes the neurotransmitter dopamine that drives the PFC
- Deep limbic system—the brain's mood control center
- Cerebellum—the area of the brain that helps coordinate thoughts

EFFECTIVELY TREATING ADD

Below I will talk about six different types of ADD and how it is important to know your type in order to get the best help. However, there are a number of treatments common to all people with ADD, for which no prescription is required.

1. Take a multiple vitamin every day. Studies have reported that they help people with learning and help prevent chronic illness. No matter what type of ADD you or your child has, take a 100 percent vitamin and mineral supplement a day. When I was in medical school, the professor who taught our course in nutrition said that if people eat a balanced diet they do not need vitamin or mineral supplements. I have seen that balanced diets are a thing of the past for many of our "fast-food families." In my experience, ADD families in particular have problems with planning and tend to eat out much more frequently than non-ADD families. Protect yourself and your children by taking a 100 percent vitamin and mineral supplement.

In a 1988 study published in the British journal *Lancet,* ninety children between the ages of twelve and thirteen were divided into three groups. One group took no tablet, one group took a typical multiple vitamin and mineral tablet, and the last group took a tablet that looked and tasted just like the vitamin and mineral tablet yet contained no vitamins or minerals. The results of this well-controlled study was that the group that took the vitamin and mineral tablet had a significant increase in nonverbal intelligence; the other two groups showed no difference at all. The subclinical vitamin and mineral deficiency may have been contributing to these students performing below their abilities.

2. Supplement your diet with omega-3 fatty acids. People with ADD have been found to have low levels of omega-3 three fatty acids in their blood, and there are three double-blind studies that indicate the value of omega-3s. Omega-3s contain two major components, EPA and DHA (docosahexaenoic acid). EPA tends to be more helpful for people with ADD. For adults, I recommend taking 2,000–4,000 mg a day; for children, 1,000–2,000 mg.

3. Eliminate caffeine and nicotine. They both interfere with sleep and decrease the effectiveness of other treatments.

4. Engage in regular exercise for forty-five minutes four times a week. Long, brisk walks do just fine.

5. Decrease television viewing, videogame playing, cell phone time, and use of other electronic devices to no more than an hour a day. This may be hard for all, but it can make a huge difference.

6. Treat food as a drug—because it is one. Most people with ADD do best when they follow the brain-healthy food program described in chapter 6. In a 2008 study from Holland, researchers found that putting children on a restricted elimination diet reduced ADD symptoms by more than 50 percent in 73 percent of children, which is basically the same effectiveness of stimulant medication without any of the side effects. Elimination diets are not easy to do. Basically, during the study, the children could only eat rice, turkey, lamb, vegetables, fruits, margarine, vegetable oil, tea, pear juice, and water. But the results were stunning. Elimination diets may be a place to start; later, other foods can be added back, which will allow you to see what items may be causing the abnormal behaviors. Working with a nutritionist may make a big difference. In this study the researchers also found that the children's moods and oppositional behaviors were improved as well.

7. Never yell at people with ADD. Many people with ADD are conflict or excitement seeking, as a means of stimulation. They can be masters at making other people mad or angry. Do not lose your temper with them. If they get you to explode, their unconscious, low-energy PFC lights up and likes it. Never let your anger be their medication. They can get addicted to it.

When you effectively treat someone with ADD, you can change their whole life. Then why are medications like Ritalin and Adderall so controversial? Because they work for some people with ADD, but they make other people much worse. Until I started doing scans I did not know why. What I found out from imaging was that ADD was not one type but could be at least six different types, and giving everyone the same treatment helped some people but created disasters in others.

Here is a brief description of the six types and treatments:

Type 1: Classic ADD—Patients exhibit primary ADD symptoms (short attention span, distractibility, disorganization, procrastination, and a lack of forward thinking) plus hyperactivity, restlessness, and impulsivity. On SPECT scans, we see decreased activity in the PFC and cerebellum, especially with concentration. Usually diagnosed earlier in life. For this type, I use stimulating supplements that boost dopamine in the brain, such as green tea,

L-tyrosine, or rhodiola or, if they are ineffective, stimulant medications (such as Adderall, Concerta, Ritalin, or Strattera). I have also found that a higher-protein, lower-simple-carbohydrate diet can be very helpful.

Type 2: Inattentive ADD—Patients exhibit primary ADD symptoms plus low energy and motivation, spaciness, and a tendency to be internally preoccupied. On SPECT scans, we see decreased activity in the PFC and cerebellum, especially with concentration. Type 2 is diagnosed later in life, if at all. It is more common in girls. These are quiet kids and adults, often labeled lazy, unmotivated, and not that smart. For this type, I use stimulating supplements that boost dopamine in the brain, such as green tea, L-tyrosine, or rhodiola or, if they are ineffective, stimulant medications (such as Adderall, Concerta, Ritalin, or Strattera). I have also found that a higher-protein, lower-simple-carbohydrate diet can be very helpful.

Type 3: Overfocused ADD—Patients exhibit primary ADD symptoms plus cognitive inflexibility, trouble shifting attention, a tendency to get stuck on negative thoughts or behaviors, a propensity for worrying and grudge holding, and a need for sameness; in addition, they tend to be argumentative and oppositional. These individuals are often seen in families with alcoholism, addiction problems, or obsessive-compulsive tendencies. On SPECT scans, we see decreased activity in the PFC with concentration plus increased anterior cingulate activity, which causes them to get stuck on negative thoughts or behaviors. Stimulants, by themselves, usually make this type worse, as people become more focused on the things that bother them. For this type, I often start with simple supplements that boost both serotonin, such as 5-HTP, and dopamine, such as green tea or L-tyrosine. If I need to use medications for this type, I generally start with Effexor, or use a combination of an SSRI, like Prozac, with a stimulant. I also recommend a diet balanced between healthy proteins and smart carbohydrates.

Type 4: Temporal Lobe ADD—Patients exhibit primary ADD symptoms plus tend to have short fuses, periods of anxiety, headaches or abdominal pain, dark thoughts, memory problems, and difficulties reading; they sometimes misinterpret comments. Often there is a history of head injury in the past or a family history of rages. On SPECT scans, we see decreased activity in the PFC with concentration and decreased temporal lobe activity. Stimulants, by themselves, usually make people with this type more irritable. In considering supplements for this type, I generally use a combination of a stimulating supplement, such as green tea or L-tyrosine, along with GABA to help calm and stabilize moods. If memory or learning is an issue, I will use green tea or L-tyrosine with memory-enhancing supplements such as ginkgo, vinpocetine, and huperzine A. If medicine is needed, I generally prescribe a combination of anticonvulsant medications (such as Neurontin) and stimulants, along with a higher protein diet.

Type 5: Limbic ADD—Patients exhibit primary ADD symptoms plus chronic mild sadness, negativity, low energy, low self-esteem, irritability, social isolation, and poor appetite and sleep patterns. On SPECT scans, we see decreased activity in the PFC at rest and with concentration and increased deep limbic activity. Stimulants, by themselves, usually cause problems with rebound or cause depressive symptoms. This type is generally effectively treated with the stimulating supplement SAMe or the stimulating antidepressant Wellbutrin. Supplement alternatives to SAMe include L-tyrosine or DL-phenylalanine.

Type 6: Ring of Fire ADD—Patients exhibit primary ADD symptoms plus extreme moodiness, anger outbursts, oppositional traits, inflexibility, fast thoughts, excessive talking, and sensitivity to sounds and lights. I refer to this type as ring of fire because of the intense ring of overactivity that I saw on the brain scans of affected people. This type is usually made much worse with stimulants if used alone. For this type, I usually start with a supplement combination of GABA, 5-HTP, and L-tyrosine. Sometimes a stimulant may also be needed. Medication alternatives include a combination of an anticonvulsant (such as Neurontin), SSRI, and a stimulant.

Knowing your type is essential to getting the right help for yourself. If these descriptions are not clear enough, consider contacting one of our clinics (www.amenclinics.com).

ADD IN INTIMATE RELATIONSHIPS

Circle the statements that apply to your intimate partner (if you have one):

1. Do you feel your partner often does not listen to you?
2. Do you often feel that you cannot trust your partner to follow through on something he or she promised to do?
3. Do you feel your partner often puts things off until the last minute?
4. Do you feel your partner often embarrasses you in front of others by thoughtless words or actions?
5. Is your partner often late or in a hurry?
6. Do you feel your partner often starts problems just for the sake of having a fight?
7. Do you feel that you're always the one chasing your partner down to talk about an important issue?

8. Does your partner often go into a rage with little or no provocation?

9. Is your partner sensitive to noise or touch?

10. Does your partner often make spur-of-the-moment decisions that he or she regrets later on?

11. Does your partner get resentful or bored with the everyday tasks of living?

12. Is your partner especially hard to get up or grumpy in the morning?

13. Does your partner have trouble verbalizing his or her intimate feelings?

If more than four statements are checked, there is a suspicion that adult ADD may be affecting your partner. Getting the right help can improve your relationship.

ADD can ruin relationships, as the following five vignettes illustrate.

STORY 1: DISTANCE AND FRUSTRATION

Rhonda was the office manager for her husband's medical practice. Samuel was a family doctor and he had a very busy practice. Samuel wanted his wife to work in the practice to protect the family assets and oversee the employees. Initially, Rhonda was happy to help, but soon she found her work to be overwhelming. She had trouble managing the office and home life. The two children (Billie, age eight, and Sarah, age five) began to act up more with both parents gone during the day. Before Rhonda went to work with Samuel, she was able to do the housework and keep some semblance of order at home. After going to work, however, she became completely disorganized. Her lack of concentration at work caused her to put in extraordinarily long hours, which left her feeling always behind and frustrated at home. Samuel saw how disorganized his wife was and offered to help. Rhonda saw his gesture as a slap in the face of her ability "to be like all of the other women who work and maintain families." Rhonda's lack of focus and follow-through caused things to slip through the cracks at work, and she became completely overwhelmed by the disorganization at home. She came to see me when she was on the verge of quitting her job and maybe even quitting her marriage. It took work with both her and her husband to get things back on track.

STORY 2: CHRONIC CONFLICT

Sally and George were very passionate about each other at first. They had a very intense relationship. After their marriage, they spent nearly every waking moment with each other in a family business. Unfortunately, they started to fight, and over time the fighting became constant. The fights were mostly over little things, but they occurred at a continual level and always included a negative word or dig said toward the other person. It seemed that there was some drive in the relationship toward turmoil. Nowhere was this more evident than on the day of an important business negotiation. Sally was the main negotiator for the business. Before most important negotiations, Sally would deliberately pick a fight with George. This caused tremendous uproar and pain. Yelling, cursing, throwing things, and threats of divorce were common events during these blow-ups. "Sally thrived on the fights," George said. "I never understood how she could go from hating me to being as cool as a cucumber during the negotiation meeting. She was a master at negotiation after fights." George also noted that without a fight Sally wasn't as calm during other business meetings. "It was like the fight was her drug," he said. The conflict seemed to make her better at work, but it was tearing apart their marriage. It was only after their marital therapist recognized that Sally suffered from ADD (and the subsequent treatment) that their marriage was able to make the turnaround that both of them so desperately wanted.

STORY 3: SPOUSAL ABUSE

There seemed to always be trouble between Bob and Beth. Even their courtship was rocky with many breakups and makeups. They met in high school, introduced by friends at a party. Both of them had used a fair amount of drugs, including marijuana and alcohol. Bob also used a significant amount of cocaine. He said it helped him study and do better at work. Both had family problems. And neither one of them were much interested in school. They got married after Beth became pregnant. Fighting became a regular part of their lives together, especially on the nights when alcohol was involved. Beth was not one to back away from a fight. In fact, her husband nicknamed her "the War Department" because, as he claimed, she seemed to frequently start fights when no problems were present. Bob admittedly had a very short fuse, and the drinking and drug use totally took away any self-control he had. On several occasions, the police were called by the neighbors who heard screaming coming from their home. After several incidents of "mutual spousal abuse," the judge ordered a psychiatric evaluation of both parties. At first, the couple laughed off the evaluation, but when the counselor made them look at their lives together (the drug abuse, constant fighting, continued underachievement, and negative impact their behavior was having on their son), they started to take the situation seriously. Both parties made significant improvements with a combination of treatments, including therapy, dietary supplements, and medication. After their rocky start, you wouldn't recognize the couple now.

STORY 4: DIVORCE

Hal and Kathy were very much in love when they first got married. They had a lot in common, were very passionate with each other, and seemed to share common goals. At first, Kathy loved Hal's spontaneity. She had some trouble loosening up, but Hal made her laugh and gave her permission to let her hair down. After several months of marriage, however, Kathy became very frustrated with Hal. He was often late coming home, forgetting to call her. He didn't finish tasks he started. He refused to pick up his own clothes or his dishes from the table. He said hurtful things to Kathy without thinking. Kathy found that she was becoming a nag. She hated the feeling. The distance between Hal and Kathy grew to the point where both of them thought of having affairs. When Hal gave in to the temptation, their marriage ended in divorce.

STORY 5: SUICIDE

John was described by his mother as "three boys in one." He was very active and mischievous as a toddler. He was tested as intellectually gifted in the second grade but by fourth grade felt bored with school. His school performance took a major nose dive after the ninth grade, and he dropped out of school in his junior year. He then entered the Marine Corps where he excelled with military structure. After he got out of the service, he married his sweetheart and started to work for the sheriff's department in his small Midwestern hometown. Because of his restlessness he started to drink too much. There were nights when he was so drunk, he would beat his wife. On two occasions, he raped her. Shortly before his wife took his newborn son and left him, he was fired from his job as a sheriff for stealing a one-ounce shot glass while he was intoxicated. After she divorced him, he married three other women. None of the relationships worked out. He drifted from job to job and could not settle down. Finally, out of desperation and chronic failure he shot and killed himself at the age of thirty-six.

ADD was a contributing factor in all of the above stories in one or both parties. These are not unusual stories. Untreated ADD often has a serious negative impact on every aspect of a female's life, whether she has it herself or someone she cares about does.

WHEN TREATMENT WORKS

I keep a notepad in my desk to write down what people tell me during their follow-up visits to the clinic. The following are actual comments from women who were treated for ADD:

> "I experienced an increased awareness of the world around me. I saw the hills for the first time when driving to work. I saw the bay when I crossed over the bridge. I actually noticed the color of the sky!"

> "I experienced a 180-degree difference in my attitude."

> "My husband said he doesn't have a knot in his stomach anymore."

> "I look at my children and say, 'Aren't they cute?' rather than complaining about them."

> "I could enjoy the moment. My thoughts are calmer, quieter, and easier to live with."

> "I could sit and watch a movie for the first time in my life."

> "I am able to handle situations where I used to be hysterical. I am able to see when I'm starting to overreact."

> "The lens on my life is much clearer."

> "I was tremendously overscheduled. No sane person would do that!"

> "It amazes me that a simple treatment can take me from wanting to jump off the bridge to loving my husband and enjoying my children."

> "It is like being given sight!"

> "I'm not running at train-wreck speed."

> "For the first time, I felt in charge of my life."

> "I'm better able to keep things in perspective."

"I used to think I was stupid. It seemed everyone else could
do more things than me. I'm starting to believe that there
may be intelligent life in my body."

"My appetite is more normal." "I'm out of the damned black
hole I was in."

"I used to be the kind of person who would go walking
by myself in downtown Detroit at 2 a.m. Now, on the
medication, I would never do something so stupid. Before,
I just wouldn't think about the consequences."

"Now I can give talks in front of groups. Before, my mind
would always go blank. I organized my life around not
speaking in public. Now my brain feels calmer, clearer."

"I feel like I think everyone else feels."

"I'm not as intimidated by others like I used to be."

"My husband may not be as happy as before I was on
treatment. Now I can think and he doesn't win all of the
arguments. I'm going to have to retrain him to not always
expect to get his way."

"I'm not losing my temper."

"It's like waking up after being asleep your whole life."

"I feel in control of my life."

"Six months ago there was no way I would drive on L.A.
freeways. Now I can drive on them with no problem."

"I can't stand useless confrontation, and I used to thrive
on it!"

WHY I AM SO PASSIONATE ABOUT HELPING FEMALES WITH ADD

On the surface, Breanne, my oldest daughter, was the perfect child.
She was always easy, always sweet, her room was always clean, and she

worked hard in school, but the truth is I never thought she was very smart. It deeply saddens me to write this, but that was how I felt. I had to teach her simple things over and over, and she did not learn her times tables until she was in fifth grade. When she was in third grade, I had her tested by a colleague, who basically told me the same thing, that she wasn't that smart. She didn't say it that way, but I could read between the lines. But the psychologist said Breanne would be okay because she worked so hard. In fact, in eighth grade Breanne won a presidential scholar award, not for academics but for effort.

In her sophomore year, however, things started to fall apart. She was in a college prep school and stayed up every night until one or two o'clock in the morning to get her homework done. Then one night, while studying biology, she came to me in tears and said she thought she could never be as smart as her friends. It broke my heart. The next day I pulled up her original brain scan from when she was eight years old. When I first started to do scans in 1991, I scanned everyone I knew. I had scanned my three kids, my mother, even myself. At the time, I only had the experience of someone who had seen fifty scans. Now, seven years later, I had seen thousands of scans. With experienced eyes, I was horrified with what I saw. Breanne had low overall activity, especially in the front part of her brain.

I came home that night and told Breanne what I saw and told her I wanted to get a new scan. Because of the injection required for the scan, she protested. "I don't want a scan, Dad. All you think about are scans." But I am a child psychiatrist. I know how to get my way with kids. I felt this was very important and so I asked her what it would take to get a scan. She told me she wanted a telephone line in her room. I started to think that maybe she was smarter than I thought. Her new SPECT study was virtually identical to the one seven years earlier. I cried when I saw it.

The next night, after giving her a low dose of medication, I rescanned her, and her brain normalized. Breanne's learning struggles had nothing to do with her intelligence. The low activity in her brain was limiting the access she had to her own brain. I put her on a low dose of medicine along with specific dietary supplements. A few days later she said that learning was much easier for her. She started bringing home A's on her tests, which had never happened before. When she went to biology class, she said she understood concepts for the first time. Usually a shy child in class, she started raising her hand, and even participated in debates. At dinner one night, she winked at me and said, "I kicked butt in a debate today." This was not the same child I knew. Four months after her scan, she got straight A's for the first time in her life. She repeated the feat all the way through high school and most of college. After college, Breanne was able to get into the University of Edinburgh, one of the best veterinarian schools in the world. She has a completely different perception of herself—one that fits her reality of being smart, competent, and able to look forward to a bright future. Even though Breanne decided not to go to the University of Edinburgh because she had just given birth to her first child, she knew she was good enough to be accepted, which made all the difference in her sense of self.

Whenever I tell Breanne's story at lectures, many women come up to me afterward with tears in their eyes and tell me that they can relate to her. If only they had known, how life would have been different for them. "You cannot change the past," I tell them, "but you can certainly start where you are now and work hard to change the future." I want *your* future to be the best it can be so that you can unleash the power of your female brain, no matter where you start from.

Hour 8 Exercise—Know Your Focus and Energy Robbers and Boosters

First, if you think you might have ADD, talk to your health care provider. As you've seen from the stories in this chapter, treating ADD will have a positive impact on every area of your life.

Even if ADD is not an issue for you, almost all of us want better energy and focus. Circle the focus and energy robbers and boosters below to see which ones apply to you. Then take steps today to lose the robbers and boost the boosters.

Focus and Energy Robbers	Focus and Energy Boosters
Any brain problems	Begin an overall brain-healthy program.
Brain trauma	Focus on brain protection.
Poor sleep	Get adequate sleep, at least seven hours a night.
Low blood sugar	Eat frequent small meals with at least some protein to maintain healthy blood sugar.
Poor diet	Begin a brain-healthy diet.
Alcohol/drug abuse	Eliminate alcohol and drugs.
Depression	Seek effective treatment for depression.
Anxiety	Meditate for relaxation.
Chronic stress	Begin a stress-reduction plan.
Lack of exercise	Exercise.
Hormone problems (e.g., thyroid, testosterone, estrogen, cortisol)	Optimize hormone levels.
Low vitamin D levels	Optimize vitamin D levels.
Medical problems, such as B_{12} deficiency	Treat any underlying medical problems.
Many medications	Take a fish oil supplement to decrease inflammation and enhance blood flow.
Diabetes	Watch your diet and begin an exercise regimen.
Environment toxins	Increase ventilation and eliminate any toxins.

Any systemic inflammation	Begin an anti-inflammation regimen, including fish oil, healthy diet, and folic acid
Chemotherapy	Take supplements, such as vitamins B_3 and B_6, L-tyrosine, DL-phenylalanine, green tea leaf extract with L-theanine, panax ginseng, rhodiola, ashwagandha, and SAMe
Excessive caffeine	Get your caffeine boost from tea, which has been shown to help keep weight off and boost exercise ability, improve muscle recovery from workouts, and improve attention span and relaxation

Do the simple 12-minute meditation described in chapter 6 (p. 000). This exercise has been found to boost blood flow to the PFC. If you can do it twelve minutes a day for eight weeks, it can strengthen your PFC.

Recite the following simple sounds known as the five primal sounds: "sa," "ta," "na," and "ma"; the vowel *a* at the end of each sound is drawn out (like "ahhhh") and is considered to be the fifth sound. The meditation involves touching the thumb of each hand to the index finger while chanting "sa," the middle finger while chanting "ta," the ring finger while chanting "na," and the pinkie finger while chanting "ma." The sounds and fingering are repeated for two minutes out loud, two minutes whispering, four minutes silently, two minutes whispering, and two minutes out loud.

9

BE BEAUTIFUL ON THE INSIDE AND OUT

STOP THE NEGATIVE CHATTER AND MAKE A PLAN TO LOOK AND FEEL AMAZING

*Focusing on inside and outside beauty together is the
ninth step to unleashing the power of the female brain.
The true beauty in a woman is reflected in her soul. It is the
caring that she lovingly gives, the passion that she shows. The
beauty of a woman grows with the passing years.*

—AUDREY HEPBURN

After a long trip, Tana and I landed at LAX, tired and ready to find our car so we could head home. Ahead of us on the Jetway was an older woman who looked confused. She was trying to ask the uniformed flight attendant for help, but the airline employee was distracted and brushed her off. Tana, seeing the fear in the elderly woman's eyes, immediately stepped in. She established eye contact and took the time to listen to her. Her husband had just died, the woman told Tana, and she came to L.A. to be with her son. She said her husband usually took care of getting them where they needed to be. Tana grabbed her arm and guided her to baggage claim to wait to meet her son. As I watched Tana take care of this woman, I thought to myself that she had never looked more beautiful. Even though most people think about beauty as a specific size, shape, or color, true beauty is about attitude, connection, and making a difference.

One day at work, I got a voice mail from a woman who was famous for her beauty. As I listened to the message, I remember catching my breath. Yet an hour after meeting her, I never thought of her as beautiful again. Her attitude, manner, and self-centeredness took away any attraction. I remember feeling odd at how fast any attraction to her I might have felt had vanished.

No doubt, being beautiful on the outside makes men pay attention to you, but if it is not consistent with beauty on the inside, it quickly fades and even turns toxic.

Likewise, I have met many women who were not stunning on the outside, but their sense of humor, passion, caring, intelligence, and the way they carried themselves made me look forward to seeing them. Their ability to attract people to them was deeper and longer lasting.

What does it mean to be beautiful? Artists, poets, and fashion designers have debated the definition of beauty since the beginning of time. If you're trying to meet the ideal of any one of them, you'll drive yourself crazy, make yourself miserable, and miss out on the most effective beauty treatment of all. That's because the best way to become your most beautiful self is to work from the inside out to nourish and nurture your unique brand of beauty. That's how you become irresistible.

None of this implies, however, that appearance on the outside is irrelevant. Ultimately, men are attracted to women who appear healthy. A man tends to be attracted to a symmetrical, fertile, healthy-looking woman. His genetic brain is looking at a woman and deciding whether or not he wants his children to carry her genes. Unconsciously, we look for signs of health, such as clear skin and bright eyes. A number of scientists believe that body symmetry also plays a critical role in our view of beauty. The theory behind this notion is that asymmetrical features give clues to underlying health problems that could yield more troubled offspring. In a study at the University of New Mexico, college males found symmetrical female faces more attractive than asymmetrical faces. In addition, women who were blessed with symmetry had a history of more sexual partners and tended to lose their virginity at an earlier age.

Having the best brain possible will help you be more beautiful on the inside and out. Did you know that the health of your skin is a reflection of the health of your brain? If you have healthy processes in your body, you will both look and function more vibrantly. Likewise, good health habits, such as sleep, great nutrition, exercise, and some simple supplements boost attractiveness; poor health habits, such as smoking, overeating, and chronic stress, make you look and feel older than you are.

FROM BODY OBSESSION TO SELF-POSSESSION

Yes, it's true that men like to look at women. We can't help it, any more than you can help looking at men. Fifty percent of both male and female brains are dedicated to vision. Before a potential partner gets to enjoy your thoughtful disposition, sense of humor, or intelligence, he sees what you look like. Whether he decides to pursue you depends on whether he likes what he sees. So you want to take care of your physical appearance.

But what he finds attractive about you may not be what you think.

Every man has a unique ideal of beauty, and it probably has nothing to do with that anorexic model on the cover of *Vogue* that many young women try to emulate. Some men like slender women, but many men prefer those who are more substantial. If you surveyed a large number of men from different cultures, you'd learn that what they consider attractive covers a wide array of shapes and sizes, hair and eye color. What men say they want includes a broad spectrum of types.

But what they say they like may be irrelevant. Research from the University of Sheffield and the University of Montpellier in France indicates that there are huge differences between how people (both men *and* women) describe their ideal partner and whom they actually select as a mate. Love and attraction has a logic of its own that can completely override our conscious ideas of beauty. What actually draws us to one another is different from what we think. And yet, more than ever we seem to be obsessed with making ourselves fit some unattainable, narrow ideal image of beauty. And in the process we may be ignoring what really counts.

To get an idea of the extent of this obsession, all you have to do is look at some of the most current statistics for plastic surgery. According to the American Society of Plastic Surgeons, in 2011, 13.8 million cosmetic procedures were performed, which was a 5 percent increase over the number of procedures in 2010. This was during a recession. There were 1.6 million surgeries, including face-lifts and breast augmentations, and 12.2 million "minimally invasive" procedures, including Botox injections, soft-tissue fillers, and laser hair removal. Altogether, this represents expenditures of $10.4 billion.

Women want to look younger, shapelier, and less hairy. And this includes teenagers ranging from ages thirteen to nineteen, who made up 2 percent of the total procedures, and women between ages twenty and twenty-nine, who accounted for close to eight hundred thousand procedures. The largest percentage of procedures involved women between ages forty and forty-five, with 6.4 million procedures—people wanting to maintain their youth or perhaps correct issues that have bothered them for years, like a bump on her nose or breasts that she feels are too small. But it must be that many of these procedures were not enough to fix "the problem." The number of patients returning for additional procedures increased by 8 percent in 2011.

So lots of work is taking place. But isn't it ironic? If you were asked to tell about the most truly beautiful women you've known in your life, the way you would describe them probably has little to do with the shape of their noses or the size of their breasts. You would more likely say things like this:

"She exuded confidence and love."

"She seemed so alive."

"She had a wonderful energy about her. She seemed so
    healthy and vibrant."

"Her eyes shone. Her skin glowed."

"She was so alert and intelligent."

"She made me feel comfortable."

"She looked so happy."

"She made me feel good about myself."

What makes a woman truly unforgettable stems from her inner qualities that are then reflected outwardly. And those qualities have their basis in the part of her body that really runs the show: her brain.

It isn't that beauty is skin deep. It's that real beauty is brain deep. A pretty face doesn't hurt, but there's more to being pretty than the size of your eyes or how full your lips are. A woman can have perfect features, but if she's angry, sneering, depressed or self-absorbed, she will not be nearly as attractive as she could be. On the other hand, a woman with irregular features and a crooked smile can be devastatingly beautiful if she has a beautiful attitude toward life.

Many years ago I watched an interview with the French actress Jeanne Moreau. She must have been in her sixties at the time. She had never had plastic surgery or any cosmetic procedures, and she definitely looked her age. But there was something so appealing about her, and yes, sexy, because she was so honest, intelligent, sensuous, and confident in the person she was. She had enormous understanding of the world and the human heart. It would be hard to say specifically what made her so beautiful. The French would say she had a quality of *je ne sais quoi*—that certain something that can never be described, explained, or fully understood but that others can sense unmistakably. That's what Jeanne Moreau had. You could tell that the interviewer felt it. He was intrigued by her.

The good news is that any woman can have those same attractive qualities. And it doesn't require any exotic treatments or expensive surgical procedures. It starts by working on your inner health instead, by developing brain-healthy habits and nurturing a beautiful attitude toward yourself and your life.

There is so much you can do, starting today, that can help you uncover the beautiful, sensuous, wildly attractive woman who is already living inside you and is just waiting to be released. In this chapter, I'll give you strategies to help your brain and body look amazing.

So this is your choice. You can spend tens of thousands of dollars on plastic surgery, which will likely just lead to more procedures. Maybe you'll be happy with the results, but there's no guarantee that you'll ever look good enough in your own eyes. And one thing you can be certain of is that it will involve a great deal of time, money, and pain. Your alternative is to work on getting your brain, mind, and body as healthy as possible. The first place to start is with your thoughts about your body.

MOST WOMEN HATE THEIR BODIES

If you are like the vast majority of women, you hate your body. In a recent *Glamour* survey of three hundred women, a whopping 97 percent of women had negative things to say about their bodies in a typical day. Their typical self descriptions included:

> "You are a fat, worthless pig."
> "You're too thin. No man is ever going to want you."
> "Ugly. Big. Gross."

Some of the survey participants reported that critical thoughts about their bodies were "fleeting." But for others the problem was more serious. They suffered from self-punishing thoughts about their bodies continually. Overall it was reported that the average woman had thirteen of these negative thoughts every day. And some women were so prone to this form of self-abuse they experienced up to one hundred such thoughts every day.

Painfully, the negativity starts early. In a University of Florida study, nearly half of girls from three to six years old thought they were fat, and nearly a third wanted to change something about their bodies. And it looks like many of them are doing something about it. A study of ten-year-old girls by the Keep It Real campaign—a joint effort between Miss Representation, the SPARK Movement, Love Social, Endangered Bodies and I Am That Girl—yielded shocking results. Up to 80 percent of them have been on at least one diet at some point in their lives.

If a guy said the awful things to you that you say to yourself, you would think he was the worst human being alive who should be punished. Yet most women continue to talk that way to themselves.

Another interesting finding from the *Glamour* study, which makes perfect sense to me, as a psychiatrist, is that if a woman was dissatisfied with her career or relationship, she was much more likely to be unhappy with her body. Any uncomfortable emotions, such as stress, loneliness, or even boredom, started to magnify the negative body image chatter.

UNBRIDLED THOUGHTS CAUSE RAMPANT FEMALE SUFFERING

Shortly after we first met, Tana and I went to a workshop given by my friend Byron Katie at Esalen in Big Sur, on the coast of north-central California. Tana is a beautiful woman on the outside and inside, and I am not saying that just because she will likely read this. It shocked me to learn of her insecurities. Toward the end of the weekend conference, Katie, as her friends call her, asked us to write down our thoughts about why we hate our bodies. With Tana's permission, I quote from what she later wrote in her journal.

From Tana's Journal

I sat with my eyes closed reclining in a cocoon of pillows, overlooking the crashing waves of the Pacific Ocean. Hearing the deep, strained voice of a woman describing the reasons she hated her body, I was abruptly jolted from my peaceful state. Her list sounded almost identical to mine.

"I hate my body because I'm too fat, I'm too old, I get sick too often, by body betrays me, I hate my thighs and my butt, I hate the skin around my eyes . . ."

Her voice sounded older than mine, and I could tell that she was heavy. I opened my eyes to see who was speaking. I was stunned. The woman speaking weighed at least 300 pounds. How could her list be exactly like mine? I felt myself becoming tense and anxious, not understanding the root of my discomfort. I was having a difficult time taking a deep breath. Trying not to let my emotions show, I closed my eyes again and focused on the sound of the waves outside. Slowly I regained my balance and began to relax.

Another woman stood up and said, "I hate my body because I am fat, dumpy, and middle-aged, and my husband left me for a younger woman." The woman was convinced that all of her problems stemmed from the fact that she wasn't pretty enough, thin enough, or able to manipulate men enough! She actually said that! While these may not be the exact words, the dialogue went something like this:

"I hate my life. I know it would be different if I could be skinny, younger, and more beautiful."

"What do you hate about your body?" said Byron Katie, a beautiful woman in her early sixties who exuded a sense of peace and joy.

"It's too fat, too old, and it sags. If I could be younger and have a hard body, my life would be different. My husband left me for a

twenty-six-year-old woman. She's skinny and beautiful. She can have any man she wants. Life is different for women like that."

"So you want to be able to have the same control over your husband that the other woman has?"

"Yes. I want to be young and beautiful and have a beautiful body so I can manipulate men."

"So you don't necessarily want him to love you because he does; you want to be able to manipulate him."

"Yes. I want to be one of those women who are beautiful and able to manipulate men and make them fall in love with me."

Daniel had been encouraging me to interact in small ways throughout the weekend and I told him he must have been smoking some of the hemp the hippies were making rope from! All weekend I had been listening to others stand up and discuss their past traumas, hang-ups, addictions, and I vacillated between envying their candor and thinking they were completely nuts to expose themselves in front of strangers.

Unexpectedly, without forethought, I found myself on my feet! It was literally as though someone was lifting me off the ground and a voice that was not mine began to speak. I was a puppet and someone else was pulling the strings. I seemed to have no choice in the matter. Trembling, I stood holding my journal in my hand. There I was in my size 2 jeans, perfectly made up, with a body fat of 16 percent. I stood facing the woman, resembling the beautiful twenty-six-year-old, manipulative woman she had been describing. Though a decade older, few people guessed my age as a result of my physical condition. Swallowing the boulder in my throat, I began to read to her from my journal with tears in my eyes, voice shaking.

"I hate my body because it is not thin enough, it is not perfect enough, it got cancer, it betrays me, and is getting old. I hate the scars I have from having cancer and from my C-section. I hate the *lines starting to form around my eyes. I hate that no matter how hard I work out, I always have a little loose skin on my abdomen from having a baby. I wake up every morning and kick my own ass in the gym regardless of how tired or sick I am, and then I stand in front of the mirror picking myself apart, looking for flaws. It's never good enough."*

I paused for a moment before looking at the woman and continuing.

"You think your life would be better if you could be a perfect size 4 and be more beautiful, whatever that means. You would just have different problems. But it's never perfect enough.

"Sometimes I've hated having so much pressure to look the way I did. There were times I wished I could go eat an entire pizza myself and not have people watching and wondering if I was going to go throw it up! Sometimes I just wanted to blend in and not be seen at all. But then if you do blend in and no one notices you, one day you go into a funk and wonder what's wrong with you because you're so used to people giving you attention all the time. You can't relax either way. Sometimes I just hate my body for getting older because I'm terrified that people won't love me or value me any longer when I can't keep this up. I'm exhausted. And by the way, my first marriage still fell apart. I still wasn't good enough."

Biting back the tears threatening to spill onto my cheeks, I turned away as I noticed every eye in the room watching me. Feeling incredibly foolish, I regretted standing. The silence in the room was magnified by the pounding in my head. I had never lost my cool and become emotional like that in front of a group. I was sure these people were judging me and thinking I was just some bubble-headed bimbo who felt sorry for myself and who was looking for attention. I was formulating an exit strategy that would draw the least attention. Fortunately it was the last hour of the final day. I planned to bolt out the door without being noticed.

It turned out that many women came up to Tana and told her what she shared was very meaningful to them. If, as a beautiful woman, she had exactly the same thoughts they had, they should accept their bodies and work on suffering less and enjoying their lives more. I was very proud of Tana, but that conference seven years ago still sticks with me. Why do almost all women hate their bodies? And what can be done about it?

Of course, the answer to the first question is not simple, and it is not just unrealistic images of thin women on television or magazine covers. The first recorded use of a corset was 2,000 BCE. As we have seen, a female's brain is busy, so many women are always thinking and worrying about what is not right with them. This is worsened by the lower serotonin levels females have compared to males, which also ramp up worry. Then take the societal pressure and the comparing women do with each other, and the negative thoughts set up a permanent residence in your brain.

The answer to the second question, what can be done about it, is more straightforward. Here are four strategies to have a younger, more beautiful brain and body.

1. FOCUS ON BOOSTING THE HEALTH OF YOUR BRAIN

With a better brain, you make better health decisions, which helps you look and feel your best. I have had many women tell me that their partners report they look years younger after just a few months on my brain-healthy program. It turns out that what is good for your brain is also good for your skin. Here are strategies that will help your brain and body look more beautiful.

Get more sleep—Sleep is one of the best beauty treatments there is. Well, consider the alternative. How do you feel after a night with not enough sleep? And how do you look? The puffy eyes. The listless expression. It's hardly an appealing picture. And there are more serious consequences as well. Your brain really

suffers from chronic sleep deprivation, and that affects everything else about you, including your thinking, your mood, and
your health. J. Christian Gillin, who studied the subject with his
team at the University of California, San Diego, says lack of sleep
can have serious effects on brain functioning. He found that on
language-based tasks, his sleep-deprived subjects' language centers shut down, even though overall their brains were very active,
leading to a lot of work with little result.

And not getting enough sleep can actually make you fat! Research from the University of Chicago has found that people who are
sleep-deprived tend to eat more simple carbohydrates than people
who have had adequate sleep. When you're sleepy, you head straight
for the cookies and candy instead of the veggies, almond butter, and
low-glycemic fruit. And it adds on the pounds. Researchers at Case
Western University tracked the weight of more than sixty-eight thousand women over a period of sixteen years. The women who slept six
hours or less per night were significantly heavier than those who slept
seven hours or more. In fact, research from England's University of
Warwick found that sleep deprivation almost doubles the risk of obesity
in adults and children. Part of the reason may lie in the higher ghrelin
levels (which stimulates appetite) and lower leptin levels (the hormone
that lets you know when you're full) in people who sleep less. This was
the finding in a Stanford University study that also found higher BMI
levels in those not getting enough sleep. Other studies have shown increased insulin resistance in the sleep deprived, leading to a greater risk
of diabetes. Diabetes negatively affects blood flow, which can make you
look older and less attractive.

So lack of sleep makes you puffy, cranky, stupid, and fat. Enough
sleep—at least seven hours a night—makes your skin glow, improves
your mood, makes you smarter, and helps you lose weight.

Remember that the next time you're tempted to force your eyes to
stay open so you can watch that old movie on TV or finish reading your

text messages. Ask yourself who you really want to be the next morning. If you want to be beautiful tomorrow, sleep tonight.

Here are a few ideas that can help:

- Maintain a regular sleep schedule.
- Create a soothing, relaxing bedtime routine.
- Avoid naps during the day.
- Reserve your bedroom for sleeping and sex. Take out the phones, computers, and video games.
- Avoid eating foods late in the day that could upset your system and disturb your sleep.
- Avoid caffeinated beverages in the late afternoon or evening. They will keep you up at night, and the next day you'll need to drink more to stay awake—and the whole cycle will begin again.

Boost Blood Flow to Your Brain and All Your Organs—Blood feeds your brain and body oxygen and nutrients and takes away toxins. It helps to keep you vibrant, healthy, and working properly. Decreased blood flow can make you look old and wrinkled. If you want to look pretty and feel sexy, you have to be aware of anything you might be doing that could be interfering with your circulation. The most obvious culprits include smoking, drinking too much caffeine, suffering from excessive stress, taking certain medications, and abusing drugs. One less obvious cause may be in the food you're eating. Trans fats, processed flours, sugar, and chemical additives can be reducing your blood flow. Plus, you may have hidden food allergies or intolerances that are adding to the problem.

Keep Moving—Physical exercise is like a natural wonder drug for your brain and body. It gets your heart to pump life-giving blood into your brain, supplying more oxygen, glucose, and nutrients that your brain needs to function at its best. The benefits of exercise are tremendous:

- It encourages the growth of new brain cells.
- It enhances cognitive ability.
- It improves your mood, calms anxiety, and helps alleviate depression.
- It fends off cognitive decline while helping to prevent, delay, and lessen the effects of dementia and Alzheimer's disease.
- It enhances the ability of insulin to prevent high blood sugar levels, reducing the risk of diabetes.
- It burns fat.
- It helps ward off osteoporosis, breast cancer, and colon cancer.
- It improves muscle tone and endurance, which lowers the risk of fall accidents.
- It reduces the symptoms of ADD.
- It improves sleep.
- It can help women better cope with hormonal issues.
- It reduces the risk of high blood pressure, stroke, and heart disease.

That's a lot of benefit just for putting aside forty-five minutes four or more times a week to get your body moving. Plus, once you get over any initial resistance, it feels great. And those positive feelings seem to spill over into other areas of your life too, and you'll find yourself making healthier choices. People who are more physically active are also more likely to eat brain-healthy foods, get more and better quality sleep, seek out health-minded social support systems, and just take better care of themselves in general.

So just get started. My exercise plan is really simple. Walk like you're late for forty-five minutes four times a week. In addition, you should lift light weights, working out each major muscle group twice a week. I never want you to hurt yourself, because it can put you out of commission for months. *My program is no pain, but lots of gain over time.* Consistent exercise will boost your circulation. Not only will your skin glow, the exercise will improve the comfort you feel in your own body and builds your confidence. And that makes you beautiful.

Balance Your Hormones—As we saw in chapter 4, a properly functioning brain and body require balanced hormones. When your hormones are optimized, you are much more likely to look and feel happy, energetic, and at the top of your game. Your skin is tighter and looks younger. When your hormones are off you can look and feel confused, irritable, tired, and unable to concentrate. For example, low thyroid hormone is often accompanied by overall decreased brain activity, leaving you irritable, depressed, and unable to think clearly. It is also associated with dry skin, which makes you look older. Low testosterone levels in women not only can reduce interest in sex, but it can also have a negative effect on memory. And, of course, the roller-coaster ride of female hormones related to PMS, and then menopause, can wreak havoc with a woman's mood, her physical well-being, and her memory and thought processes. Food cravings and weight issues also go hand in hand with hormones that are out of whack.

More Sex?—You are thinking, "Of course a guy would think that," but the research also backs it up. Sexual activity can boost hormones like estrogen and DHEA, and that can promote smoother, tighter skin. Sex also increases levels of oxytocin, the bonding and trust hormone, and decreases levels of the stress hormone cortisol. Not only does this feel good immediately, but tests of longevity in men show that greater frequency of orgasm is associated with increased life span. And women who have regular sex have been shown to have significantly higher levels of estrogen in their blood compared to women with infrequent or no sex. Estrogen helps maintain a healthy cardiovascular system, reduces bad cholesterol, and increases good cholesterol and bone density and enhances skin. It also is beneficial to brain function.

Another hormone that spikes during orgasm is DHEA, which is believed to improve brain function, balance the immune system, and help maintain and repair tissue while it promotes healthy skin. It may also have a positive effect on cardiovascular health. Testosterone is also increased through regular sexual activity. Testosterone helps strengthen bones and muscles, and it offers many benefits to the brain and the cardiovascular system.

Don't forget that sexual activity is great exercise and burns calories. And the release that comes with orgasm can have a calming, sedative effect. It's often followed by great sleep. All of this can be a wonderful beauty treatment. According to research by David Weeks, a clinical neuropsychologist at the Royal Edinburgh Hospital, engaging in intercourse three times a week in a stress-free relationship can make you look ten years younger. So don't say no to loving sex in a safe relationship. It can improve your brain and make you look great!

Hydrate—To be beautiful, you need to keep yourself hydrated. That's what keeps your skin plump and juicy and youthful appearing. Good hydration helps prevent wrinkles and fine lines. And it goes deeper than that. Your body is 70 percent water, and your brain is 80 percent water. When you aren't drinking as much water as you should, your brain function is reduced. And even a little bit of dehydration will cause your body to release stress hormones. That makes you irritable and reduces your ability to think clearly. Over time, elevated levels of stress hormones can lead to memory problems and obesity. You'd never think it, but your bad mood and confusion can be due to something as unexpected as not stopping for thirty seconds to drink something. Waiting until you're so thirsty you can't ignore it any more is waiting too long. If you feel thirsty, you're already dehydrated.

Get Some Sun, but Don't Get Overexposed—The sun is necessary for life on earth, but too much can do a number on your skin. That's especially true today when a thinning ozone layer means that more of the sun's harmful rays are reaching us on the ground. Some sun is a good thing and promotes healthy skin by boosting the vitamin D levels in your body. But too much sun can lead to premature aging and brown spots. Try to achieve the right balance by getting no more than thirty minutes of sun exposure during the day. If you're going to be out any longer, protect yourself with clothing or sunscreen. But be careful with sunscreen as it can have toxic chemicals. I recommend plant-based natural sunscreens with zinc oxide.

Supplements to Pamper Your Brain and Skin—Certain supplements can boost your brain and skin at the same time. Here are some of the ones I recommend:

- *Vitamin D:* This is an essential nutrient for your brain and your skin. Low levels are associated with depression and memory problems, and problems with your skin like psoriasis. Get your vitamin D level optimized.
- *Fish oil:* This supplement is great for your brain, heart, skin, and your hair. One way it keeps your skin looking younger and more vibrant is through its anti-inflammatory properties. The typical dosage is 1–2 g a day for health maintenance. I recommend higher dosages to support healing.

- *Evening primrose oil:* This supplement is often taken by women who are facing hormone issues. But it also contains GLA, an essential fatty acid. Scientific evidence indicates that GLA can help support healthy skin.
- *DMAE:* Also known as deanol, this analog of the B vitamin choline is a precursor of the neurotransmitter of acetylcholine. Research shows it has anti-aging properties that diminish wrinkles and improve the appearance of skin. A 3 percent DMAE facial gel has been found to be effective in mitigating forehead wrinkles and fine lines around the eyes. It also improved lip shape, fullness, and the overall appearance of skin. These positive effects seem to be maintained even after treatment stops. In addition, DMAE has been shown to have anti-inflammatory effects; it increases skin firmness and improves facial muscle tone. It may also help improve the appearance of age spots. The typical recommended dosage is 300–500 mg daily.
- *Phenylalanine:* This amino acid has been shown to help support mood and pain control. It may also help with a skin condition called vitiligo, that causes white patches of skin as the cells responsible for skin pigmentation die or lose their ability to function.
- *Alpha-lipoic acid:* Alpha-lipoic acid (ALA) is naturally in the body and may protect against cell damage under a number of conditions. Research shows that a cream containing 5 percent ALA was associated with significant improvement in facial skin aging. The typical dose recommended for adults is 100 mg twice a day.
- *Grape seed extract:* When wine and grape juice are processed, grape seeds are cast off as a waste product. An extract made from those seeds may be a magic elixir for your skin and brain. Grape seeds contain flavonoids and oligomeric

proanthocyanidins (OPCs). OPCs have been shown to have antioxidant power that is twenty times greater than vitamin E and fifty times greater than vitamin C. Grape seed extract has the antioxidant effect of bonding with collagen, which promotes youthful skin, elasticity, and flexibility. It also seems to improve brain function while decreasing the beta-amyloid plaques that are associated with Alzheimer's disease. In other research, proanthocyanidins have been shown to help protect the body from sun damage. It also improves blood circulation by strengthening capillaries, arteries, and veins. There is also strong scientific evidence that it can help with skin edema, venous insufficiency, and varicose veins. The typical adult dose of grape seed extract is 50–100 mg daily.

2. CORRECT THE ANTS ABOUT YOUR APPEARANCE BY WRITING THEM DOWN AND TALKING BACK TO THEM

Byron Katie's four-question technique, discussed in chapter 6, is very powerful in helping you make peace with your appearance.

. Here are two examples from patients. The first one was in her mid thirties, single, and about 30 pounds overweight.

ANT: You are a fat, worthless pig.

Is it true? "No, obviously, I am not worthless or a pig."

Can you absolutely know that it is true? "No."

How do you feel when you believe the thought? "Terrible, worthless, like no one will ever want me. I hate myself and want to be someone else. I then start to overeat chips, cookies, and ice cream as a way to soothe the anxiety and the depression and hopelessness I feel."

Who would you be or how would you feel without the thought? "So much better, happier, less self-critical."

Turn the thought around. "I am not a fat, worthless pig. I have worth in so many areas . . . work, family, spiritually. It is true I need to work on getting healthier, that is true, but abusing myself has not and will not be helpful."

The following patient was a sixty-two-year-old divorced woman who wanted to start Internet dating.

ANT: I am old and no one will want me.

Is it true? "Yes. I have not dated in decades and no one will want to see my old naked body."

Can you absolutely know that it is true? "No. Of course, I cannot know that for sure."

How do you feel when you believe the thought? "Lonely, ugly, and I hate myself. I get depressed and withdrawn."

Who would you be or how would you feel without the thought? "I would feel excited about the potential of meeting someone new, someone to have fun with. But if I am so negative, no one will have fun with me. I don't have fun being with me."

Turn the thought around. "I am young and someone will want me. Actually, people in my family tend to live into their eighties and nineties. If I take care of myself, I can live thirty more years. It is time to get healthy and meet someone fun."

3. GET THE STRESS OUT OF YOUR EYES AND SKIN

Your skin is the brain on the outside. Numerous studies have shown that when you experience psychological stress, your brain responds by sending signals to your skin to react as if it is under physical attack. This can result in a rash, flushing, blushing, or an increase in the production of protective oils and a decrease in the skin's less-critical functions, such as hair growth. More oil and less hair growth typically equals more blemishes and thinning hair. If you are stressed out about your new job, a test, or a big date, your skin is more likely to break out.

The brain–skin connection is so strong that some people have begun calling the skin "the brain on the outside." In fact, the skin has been found to produce many of the same neuropeptides—including melatonin, serotonin, cortisol—used by the brain. It is clear that the health and appearance of your skin are a reflection of the health of your brain.

There's nothing attractive about a wrinkled brow, the nervous darting of anxious eyes, or the ring of dangerous belly fat caused by emotional overeating and too many stress hormones circulating in your blood. And here again, the effects go deeper than you can see. Chronic stress constricts blood flow to your brain. That lowers overall brain function, impairs memory, and causes your brain to age prematurely. Decreased activity in your hippocampus, amygdala, and the PFC upsets both your cognitive function and your emotional balance.

Chronic stress also directly affects the way you look by causing your skin to lose collagen and elastin, two proteins that add support and elasticity to give your face that youthful, firm appearance. The result is sagging skin and wrinkles. In a cruel twist of fate, at the same time it can upset your hormones and lead to adult acne.

If you want to look younger and enjoy your life more, it's critical that you calm your stress. And that means paying attention to yourself. When things go wrong in our lives, we tend to look outward to fix or complain about the problem. We don't realize that the way we see the situation, and how we respond to it emotionally, is a big part of the problem. When we start putting our attention back on ourselves we can calm the stress reaction, and that actually changes the situation. See chapter 6 for ways to soothe the female brain.

WHAT HURTS YOUR SKIN—
AND WHAT MAKES IT BEAUTIFUL

Skin Damagers	Skin Enhancers
Too much caffeine	Limit caffeine intake.
Alcohol	Restrict alcohol consumption.
Smoking	Quit immediately.
Poor diet	Embark on a brain-healthy diet.
Too much sugar	Reduce sugar intake.
Yo-yo dieting	Maintain stable weight.
Dehydration	Drink plenty of water (half your weight in ounces every day for people under 250 pounds).
Lack of sleep	Get adequate sleep, at least seven hours per night.
Lack of exercise	Engage in physical activity at least four days a week.
Chronic stress	Meditate and practice deep-breathing exercises.
PTSD	Seek therapy.
Hormonal imbalances	Balance hormones.
Thyroid conditions	Balance thyroid levels.
Psychiatric conditions	Seek appropriate treatment, such as therapy and medication.
Memory problems	Practice brain-healthy habits or seek treatment, such as medication.
Sun exposure	Limit sun exposure to twenty minutes before applying sunscreen.
Aging	Supplement with vitamin D, fish oil, DMAE, phenylaline, ALA, and grape seed.

4. YOU WILL BE MORE BEAUTIFUL WHEN YOU SEE THE BEAUTIFUL IN LIFE

Spend time focusing on the things you are grateful for in your life. It will actually make your brain work better and make your eyes and smile brighter! After decades of social psychology research, Dr. Martin Seligman at the University of Pennsylvania believes that happiness can be cultivated. It starts by focusing on what is right in your life. He reported that if his research subjects wrote down three things they were grateful for every day, they would notice a significant boost in their level of happiness in just three weeks. If you do this exercise on a daily basis, you will not only feel better but also look prettier and be more fun to be around.

If you have been suffering because you think you are not pretty enough or not good enough, reconsider your thoughts and ideas about what is beautiful. The harmful habits and wrong ideas that have been ingrained into you since you were a child may be preventing you from fully living the beauty that is your essential nature. You were born to be beautiful, inside and out. How you live physically and emotionally will determine if you leave someone wanting more of you, or less.

Hour 9 Exercise—Get a Massage and Enjoy a Sauna

Taking time to relax and care for your body is essential to looking and feeling beautiful. Get a relaxing massage to loosen up your muscles and then spend fifteen minutes in an infrared sauna, which has been shown to increase circulation; lower blood pressure; increase the workload on the heart at the rate of a brisk walk; and help with relief of pain, chronic fatigue, weight, and addictions. During a sauna, blood flow increases to the skin, which brings nutrients to subcutaneous and surface skin tissue, helping to keep your skin healthy. The increased sweat gland activity helps to remove toxins. If you cannot find an infrared sauna, a regular one is the next best.

10

UNDERSTAND SEX AND THE FEMALE BRAIN

OPTIMIZE YOUR BRAIN FOR GREATER PLEASURE, DEEPER RELATIONSHIPS, AND LASTING LOVE

Boosting your brain for lasting connections is the tenth step to unleashing the power of the female brain. The female brain is the largest and most important sex organ in the universe.

Sweetheart. *Babe. Hon. I love you.* These are the words we all long to hear, that we all long to say—and mean them! We say them from the bottom of our hearts and to hear them makes our hearts sing. Oops. I should have said *brains* instead of *hearts*. It's our brains that light up and send rewarding hormones throughout our bodies when we hear those magic phrases. And it is our brains, not our hearts, that break when love is lost.

If you want more love in your life, you should be paying attention to your brain. As a woman, you have a whole system built right into your physiology that is designed to prepare you to love and be loved and to have thrilling, fulfilling relationships. Everything you do to cooperate with that system by keeping your brain healthy and your hormones in balance will help you love more and be more loved. Then nature will take its course, and you will have amazing connections.

Here are the facts you can use to optimize your brain and invigorate your love life.

THE STORY OF LOVE

ACT 1: LUST

If you've ever been in love, you know that there are different kinds of love, and the kind you feel can change over the course of a relationship. What you may not know is that each kind of love is guided by its own brain system and involves a different set of hormones and neurotransmitters.

Dr. Helen Fisher, an anthropologist from Rutgers University, has been researching the subject for years and is one of our prime authorities on it. She identifies three different kinds of love, along with the specific brain correlates and system of hormones and neurotransmitters that go with each. These three kinds of love all occur within one relationship, at different stages.

The first type of love is lust—the kind of bodice-ripping passion you feel when you first notice that handsome stranger staring at you across the room, or that man in the office you've been working alongside for six months, but whom you suddenly see very differently as you watch him come back all sweaty from his lunchtime workout at the gym.

According to research by Syracuse University professor Stephanie Ortigue, that process of falling in love takes about a fifth of a second and involves twelve different brain areas. Under the powerful driving force of androgens and estrogens, you feel an intense desire for sexual gratification with that individual. Other feel-good chemicals that add to the party are dopamine, oxytocin, adrenaline, and vasopressin. It's a very heady combination that makes you feel thunderstruck, and it actually affects you cognitively. The world really does look different to you.

And that man you're lusting after? You can't even see his flaws. He's bathed in the same glow that surrounds the heroes on the covers of romance novels.

The part of your brain that's primarily involved in all this is your hypothalamus, which also controls your other physical needs, like hunger and thirst. And the drive for sexual union is just as powerful. It has to be. It's what makes the human species survive!

ACT 2: ROMANCE

In most species of animals, lust has its way, mating occurs, and the two individuals go their separate ways. But for humans it's very different. The initial attraction is the trigger that leads into one of the most wonderful and sought after experiences of life: romance.

This is the passionate, all-consuming emotion that makes you feel on top of the world when everything is going well, and it throws you into the depths of despair when love is thwarted, unrequited, or rejected. It is for romance that lovers swim across oceans, scale mountains, and slay dragons to impress, delight, or simply be with the beloved. According to Dr. Fisher, it's more powerful than lust. People don't kill themselves for sex—but they will for a broken romance.

In fact, Dr. Fisher says that love is not just a feeling. It's actually a goal-directed drive that affects our behavior and thinking by improving performance where the lover is involved. In one of Ortigue's studies, subliminal exposure of the beloved's name during a decision task dramatically improved the performance of her women subjects who were in love. The women may have been sleepless, fluttery, and unable to concentrate on other things, but anything related to their beloved made them very attentive indeed.

Brain imaging studies of subjects in the early stages of this kind of crazy love shows very high activity in the ventral tegmental area and the nucleus accumbens. These, it turns out, are the centers of reward that are activated when a person inhales cocaine. In lovers, these areas are bathed in dopamine, which drives us to attain the reward we've fixed our aim on. Other chemicals that are elevated and related to stress and excitement generally are cortisol, phenylephrine, and norepinephrine. By the way, phenylephrine is also found in chocolate, which is why chocolate is related to love and why eating it is a common source of solace to the love-starved.

Once you're hooked like this, even the sight of his belongings makes the atmosphere electric. As you drive into the parking lot at work, you search eagerly for his car. And when you see it, the area takes on a quality of interest, importance, and excitement that is in sharp contrast to the drabness of every other part of the world. There is no place else where you want to be.

While all this is going on, the neurotransmitter serotonin is at low levels. Low serotonin is also related to obsessive thinking, which is certainly a common symptom of this kind of love, where you can't get that person out of your mind.

ACT 3: AFFECTION AND LONG-TERM COMMITMENT

No one can stay madly in love forever. You'd exhaust yourself and never get anything else done. Plus, if a child results from all this excitement, another set of hormones kicks in to prepare you to take care of this new responsibility—hormones that are also driven by the survival needs of the species.

No, you can't stay madly in love indefinitely, but another kind of love develops that is also under the guidance of your brain and your hormones. The switch-over seems to come somewhere between eighteen months and four years of the relationship. Once again, the hypothalamus becomes important, but the hormones involved now are oxytocin and vasopressin, and these lead to bonding and a sense of belonging. All the love hormones have to strike the right balance, and here is a perfect example. Oxytocin and vasopressin are thought to interfere with the pathways for dopamine and norepinephrine, and vice versa.

But when mad love passes, and dopamine and norepinephrine are suppressed, the bonding chemicals start coming more into play, helping ensure the continuation and evolution of the relationship.

Testosterone also interferes with oxytocin and vasopressin secretion. In fact, studies have shown that men with higher levels of testosterone marry less frequently, have a greater tendency to divorce, and can be more abusive in relationships. It may come in handy to remember that men with higher testosterone tend to have ring fingers that are longer than their index fingers. If you want to know if a potential mate is a good bet for a long-term relationship, look at his hands!

WIRED FOR LOVE

The brains of people in love light up when they look at pictures of their beloved. Dr. Fisher confirmed this in MRI studies of men and women who were in the throes of early love. But when she compared her male subjects to her female subjects, she discovered some very interesting differences.

The men showed most of their activity in parts of the brain associated with the integration of visual stimuli. These were parts of the visual cortex and visual processing areas, some of which were directly related to sexual arousal. For men, visual stimuli are very important for arousal. They are always assessing the attractiveness of females as their primary impression of them. Women sense this and spend a great deal of effort to make themselves visually appealing. Also, it's no surprise that men are much more interested in pornography than women. Those visual stimuli really get their juices flowing.

But for women, it's very different. For the women in her study, Fisher found that looking at the picture of the men they loved caused comparatively more activity in the caudate nucleus. This is an area of the brain that is involved with memory, emotion, and attention. Other areas that lit up were the septum, which is sometimes called the brain's pleasure center, and the posterior parietal cortex, which is associated with producing mental images. In addition, parts of the brain involved with memory recall were also activated.

So men are more visually oriented in sizing up a potential mate, and they are more likely to fall in love at first sight. From an evolutionary perspective, they're looking for a healthy-looking woman to bear their babies, and at this point, they're not thinking much beyond getting their seed planted.

But from the very beginning, a woman is integrating the image of her beloved into areas of her brain associated with memory. Women seem more likely to remember events in a courtship, and they may never forget that first fight and all the details of who said what. Again, this could give her an evolutionary advantage. It's not enough that her suitor is good looking. She's not just looking for one night of passionate love. She's looking for someone who will stay with her and help her raise their young. So it's very important that she remember all the details of her interactions with him. Has he demonstrated a helping attitude? Does he seem to be loyal? Does he like her family and do they like him? She's always picking up on cues that reveal his character. And she remembers all of it. Plus, she remembers the events along with the emotional content of the moment. This makes for very powerful memories that bond her to the person she loves right in the very fiber of her brain.

So, while he may be quicker to fall in love, she will be ready to commit herself to the relationship and start thinking about a future together much sooner.

What this means for you is that in the early stages of your relationship, the man in your life may overwhelm you with his passion. Every time he sees you, he'll get turned on all over again. But that doesn't mean he has the same ideas about a committed future that you're already beginning to form as you build a structure of emotional memories. As long as you understand him, you won't misread his cues and think he's ready for more than he may be. And you can be patient.

Eventually his oxytocin and vasopressin will kick in and you will both have the same goals.

THE BIG O

The French have an expression for it (of course): *le petit mort,* "the little death." Shakespeare referred to it as "die in thy lap." *It* is achieving orgasm, that amazing, convulsive release that is the climax of sexual intercourse. The center of all the sensation you feel is in your genital area, from whence it radiates throughout your body; but, in fact, its origin is in your brain. And sex researchers who have studied the brain during orgasm have found that it's not inaccurate to call it a little death—especially for women.

Researcher Barry Komisaruk of Rutgers University has found that the subjective experience of orgasm is very similar for men and women. But more recent work from the Netherlands shows that what happens in the brain is very different. Dutch neuroscientist Gert Holstege used positron emission tomography scans to study what was going in the brains of men versus women during orgasm. In men, the part of the brain that was most highly activated was the ventral tegmental area, which, as it turns out, is responsible for releasing dopamine. As you'll recall, dopamine is a neurotransmitter that is part of the brain's reward circuit and is integral to the pleasure felt by cocaine and heroin users. In fact, while this part of the brain is related to orgasmic pleasure felt by drug users, it may be the overstimulation of this part of the brain by addicts through their drug use that leads to suppressed sexual drive.

When Holstege studied his women subjects, however, he was in for a surprise. To a much greater degree than in the men, the women's brains went strangely silent during orgasm. Specifically, the left lateral orbitofrontal cortex and the dorsomedial PFC seemed to be deactivated. These parts of the brain are involved in self-control and social judgment. He also found more greatly suppressed activity in the amygdala, so there was an even greater reduction in vigilance and emotion compared to the men. Holstege concluded, "At the moment of orgasm, women do not have any emotional feelings." They completely abandon themselves to the sensation in their bodies.

Other research has found that in women during sex, there is decreased activity in the amygdala and hippocampus. These are areas associated with fear and anxiety. It seems that during sex a woman's brain suppresses these negative emotions so she can feel safe and relaxed, both necessary conditions for her to release into orgasm. Interestingly, areas of the cortex associated with pain are also activated, which means there appears to be an association between pain and pleasure in the woman, partially explaining some sadomasochistic practices. Professor Komisaruk explains that orgasm (as opposed to sex) can block pain signals. In his research with both laboratory animals and humans, he found that orgasm can inhibit the release of pain transmitters from the spinal cord. As a result, the signals can't reach the neurons in the brain that are activated in response to pain.

Oxytocin is also released in the brains of both men and women during and after orgasm. It is believed that this builds bonding and trust, and therefore it's not surprising that many a male, who would not say it at another time, will say "I love you" during or right after intercourse. Some women sense this and don't trust an "I love you" spoken during sex. She wants to hear it while they're taking a walk or eating dinner.

HOW TO HAVE BETTER ORGASMS

If you want to have better orgasms (and who doesn't?), or you have problems reaching orgasm at all, there are some things you can do to help you enjoy a more intense experience.

Love Your Partner—Researchers at the University of Geneva and the University of Santa Barbara have found evidence for what we all suspect is true: The more a woman loves her partner, the more easily she reaches orgasm and the more intense it is. Not only is this what women self-report, but when their brains were studied through magnetic resonance imaging (MRI) scans while they were being presented with the names of their lovers, the more love the women reported, the greater activity there was in the left angular gyrus, an area related to memory and emotion. They also had more activity in an area of the left-brain hemisphere responsible for addiction. So it appears that for women, love is a great aphrodisiac.

Make Sure Your Feet Are Warm—For a woman to relax enough to have an orgasm, it's necessary for her to feel safe and comfortable, and having warm feet is a big part of that. According to the researchers from the University of Groningen, having warm feet increases a woman's chance of having an orgasm by 30 percent. Possibly that's because the area of your brain concerned with sensation in your feet is located right next door to the area concerned with sensation in your genitals (this might help explain foot fetishes in some). So if your partner wants you to be more open to sex and more likely to climax, suggest that he massage your feet as part of foreplay. Even better, have him do it with some warming gel. That should help get both of you in the mood.

And while you're at it, have him kiss you on the right side of your neck or spine. (And you can try it on him too.) It is much more arousing than a kiss on the left side.

Focus Your Attention—Compared to a man, as a woman you have a special power when it comes to orgasm. Many women are able to bring themselves to orgasm just by thinking, without any physical stimulation at all. Komisaruk's research may have explained why. He found that when women thought about a part of their body being stimulated—a finger, a toe, a nipple, or their clitoris—the corresponding part of the sensory cortex of their brain would be activated, just as if they were actually being touched. This is a pretty powerful ability, and you can possibly use this information to increase your pleasure during sex if you are having trouble becoming aroused. Instead of thinking about your grocery list or your schedule the next day, bring your attention back into the moment and think about the building sensation in your clitoris. Focus on it and you can intensify what you're feeling. A little bit of imagination could result in a very real increase in pleasure.

Breathe Deeply—There are certain smells that are more likely to turn you on. And it differs for every woman. A man's musky odor can make some women swoon. But others may find it objectionable. Determine the smell that is most erotic to you, and then find a way to make your man wear it. It might be a cologne you like or the smell of fresh laundry. Many women grow weak at the scent of baby powder. If that's you, put a little on him after you shower together, and breathe in deeply.

Kiss—There's a reason women need foreplay. It takes longer for you to get aroused, and you have to be brought to a peak of excitement closer to your lover's if intercourse is going to be pleasurable for you. Kissing is a very important part of the process. Your lips are extremely sensitive and packed with nerve endings. They have one hundred times more nerve endings than your fingertips have. When you kiss, multiple mechanisms in the brain are triggered, which in turn release the chemicals of love that relax you, reduce your levels of anxiety, and make you much more receptive as the intensity of lovemaking proceeds.

Tell Him What You Want—In case you haven't noticed it, he can't read your mind. And if you stay passive in your lovemaking, he will never know what to do or what you're craving. He wants to please you, but to him, your body is a mystery. He can only go by what pleases him, but that's not much of a guide to what actually works for you. And he has no idea of his own strength. What seems to him like a gentle touch may in fact be far too intense to cause you anything but discomfort. So tell him what you want. Guide his hand. Say to him, "It feels so good when you _____," and then you fill in the blank. Then be prepared to tell him again. And again. He may not remember, and it's not because he doesn't care about you. It's because he's a man and has a sleepier brain. So don't get mad because he's not listening to you. Be patient and remind him what you like. Eventually he'll get it. And taking a more active role in your lovemaking will not only increase the sexual pleasure for both of you, but it will strengthen and deepen your relationship too.

Talk to Your Doctor—If you are on an antidepressant drug like Lexapro, Celexa, Zoloft, Prozac, or Paxil, it may be interfering with your ability to orgasm. This class of drugs boosts serotonin, which suppresses the production of dopamine, the hormone that is so essential to achieving orgasm. Your doctor may be able to switch your medication (Wellbutrin, for example, is a more stimulating antidepressant) or adjust your dosage or use other strategies, such as "taking a drug holiday" if you know that sex is going to happen during a certain time. Ginkgo or ginseng can also be helpful.

And if sex is painful, see your gynecologist. He or she can see if anything is wrong and can help you by perhaps prescribing a hormone cream or other medication.

WHEN LOVE MAKES YOU CRAZY

Unrequited love can be a killer—literally. Love can turn people into stalkers. It can make them commit suicide or homicide. It can make them grieve a lost love without respite.

In short, love can make you crazy. And the reason is the cocktail of neurotransmitters (especially dopamine) and hormones that make you react to love like a hit of cocaine and make you suffer its withdrawal like a junkie who's been denied a fix. According to Dr. Fisher, studies show that 40 percent of rejected lovers become clinically depressed—at least for a while.

Much like Fisher's work, researchers Andreas Bartels and Semir Zeki used functional MRI (fMRI) scans to look at the brains of people in love as they looked at pictures of the ones they loved and pictures of acquaintances. Like Fisher, they found that when subjects looked at the object of their romantic attachment, brain activity increased in areas associated with happiness. At the same time, there was less activity in parts of the PFC and in areas associated with fear, sadness, and depression. It seems that people in love have a brain that makes them happy and stupid. It was especially interesting that some of the areas that lit up had high concentrations of dopamine receptors. These brain areas are generally associated with addiction to drugs like heroin and cocaine. The authors noted the "potentially close neural link between romantic love and euphoric states." Of course, the similarity between love and addiction, with their cravings, single-mindedness, and symptoms of withdrawal, has long been noted by scientists and nonscientists alike.

While being happily in love makes us crazy, it's the withdrawal symptoms of rejected love that can make us crazy and dangerous. It can lead to clinical depression and sometimes violent behavior. Fisher and her colleagues studied the fMRI scans of people suffering over rejection of their love as they looked at pictures of the rejecter. They found activation of areas associated with gains and losses, craving, and regulation of emotion. Activation of the forebrain was similar to that seen in cocaine craving and addiction and may explain the obsessive behaviors associated with being rejected in love.

And we now have scientific evidence that proves that love hurts. Research at the University of Michigan shows that people suffering over a romantic breakup have brain areas activated that are the same areas involved in feeling physical pain.

Anyone who has ever been through a breakup knows how distressing it can be. Your thinking becomes obsessively focused on the person who rejected you. You can't think of anything else. And it hurts physically. You're going through the symptoms of withdrawal that are akin to what you'd be feeling if you were a drug addict trying to quit cocaine.

Now's the time to take care of your brain by following all the brain-healthy methods we've been talking about. And try to remember that the pain you're feeling is largely the result of chemicals rushing through your brain but that eventually everything will balance out again. It won't be long before you realize he wasn't right for you in so many ways, and you probably were aware of that all along.

You can even help the healing process by making a list of all the things you didn't like about him and all the little signs you'd been ignoring while you were trying to convince yourself that he was the one.

As a woman, you have tremendous powers of love and commitment and willingness to sacrifice for others. Yes, a broken heart hurts. But it's better than having no heart. Every heartbreak can lead to greater understanding and compassion, and that can be very attractive to the right person.

THE POWER OF LOVE

Love feels good. Not only that, it's good for you. Love has the power to keep you healthy, both physically and mentally. Let us count the ways.

Love Reduces Stress and Improves Well-Being—Love and sex, like other behaviors that are necessary for species survival, involve naturally rewarding and enjoyable activities. They involve feelings of well-being with stress-reducing and health-promoting potential. The effects of pleasurable experiences on the brain may inhibit activity in areas normally related to the production of anxiety, so you just feel happier and more relaxed.

The release of oxytocin and endorphins during and after orgasm has a tremendously calming and relaxing effect. That's why you sleep so well after sex. It's as though you took a sedative. And after a good night's sleep, you just feel better and less stressed the next day.

Love Reduces Negative Emotions—You know that when you're in love, little things don't bother you like they normally do. You're much more tolerant of that annoying kid behind the cash register at the grocery store. Even your mother doesn't bother you as much as she usually does. There's a reason for it. Being in love reduces your autonomic reactivity in the face of negative emotion, and the source of this new openness to the daily experiences of life involves the vagus nerve—a nerve that runs from your head through the trunk of your body. Research indicates that regulation of the vagus nerve is one of the ways in which love reduces stress and promotes well-being.

If you have a tendency to become depressed, be aware that orgasms can have an antidepressant effect. Semen itself contains chemicals like prostaglandins and fatty acids that a woman absorbs through her vagina, which can modulate her hormones and moods.

Builds Your Brain—As we get older, we lose brain cells. According to research at Princeton University, however, sexual activity may actually help us grow new brain cells. At least in studies of mice, sex is associated with the growth of brain cells in the hippocampus, one of the main memory centers of the brain. So, while stress and depression reduce cells in this area, sex seems to stimulate growth.

There is also evidence that people who are sexually active as they grow older are less likely to develop dementia. Barry Komisaruk thinks this may be related to increased blood flow to the brain and the associated higher oxygen levels. Komisaruk says that MRI scans indicate that brain neurons are more active during orgasm and use more oxygen. Oxygenated blood brings fresh nutrients to the area, keeping it healthy, nourished, and growing.

Having sex can boost brain power in another way too. Orgasm increases levels of estrogen and testosterone, both of which are good for your brain. Testosterone benefits concentration and reaction times, as does estrogen.

Makes You Healthier—More sex is related to greater longevity, boosted immunity, and fewer sick days. It can enhance your fertility, regulate your menstrual cycle, and relieve menstrual cramps. Putting more youth-inducing hormones into your blood, like DHEA, estrogen, and testosterone can benefit your cardiovascular system, lower your cholesterol, increase your bone density, and give you smoother skin.

When you engage in sex, you trigger the production of a human growth hormone that helps keep you looking younger, and all that activity keeps your blood circulating, especially to the skin. Sex is a toning, calorie-burning exercise that keeps you fit and helps you keep your weight under control. According to research at the Royal Edinburgh Hospital, having sex regularly (three times a week) can make you look up to ten years younger!

And there are additional benefits. Orgasm can help alleviate certain types of pain. This is due to the surge in oxytocin, which, in turn, releases endorphins; these are natural pain reducers. Moreover, estrogen can help relieve the pain of PMS. Even migraines can be helped. Research with migraine sufferers shows that having an orgasm can alleviate, and in some cases completely eliminate, migraine pain. So, rather than using a headache as an excuse *not* to have sex, you may want to use it as an excuse *to* have sex. The results are immediate: It costs nothing, there are fewer side effects, and you and your partner can both enjoy it.

GETTING READY FOR LOVE

Getting ready for love means more than picking out the right outfit to wear and applying a new color of lipstick. The most important beauty regimen you should be thinking about is getting your brain in order. When your brain works right, you work right. You can be loving, thoughtful, attentive, consistent, romantic, and playful. But there are many "brain issues," like ADD and depression, that can get in the way of great sex and satisfying relationships.

If you are having problems in the bedroom, it may be a good idea to look at the other aspects of your life and take care of those first.

For example, if you're riding the PMS roller coaster every month, or going through perimenopause or menopause, you may want to look into balancing your hormones, discussed earlier.

Being out of shape and overweight can interfere with your energy level and body image and, therefore, your enjoyment of sex. Get on a program of healthy eating and exercise, and take brain-healthy supplements, like fish oil. You may be surprised how your interest in sex grows as your BMI goes down.

Untreated brain trauma may be causing a variety of symptoms from inability to concentrate to anxiety, confusion, forgetfulness, and promiscuity—all of which can interfere with bonding and being a caring, reliable partner. If you suspect you are suffering from brain trauma owing to injury or toxic exposure, have it checked out. There are a variety of treatments available that can get your brain back into shape.

Drug and alcohol abuse are relationship killers. And it all starts with their negative effect on brain function. If you take illegal drugs, or even many legal ones, such as alcohol or prescribed painkillers or benzodiazepines, they will have a negative effect on your relationships. You may be medicating yourself with drugs and alcohol to dull the pain of your life, but they are actually increasing the pain and preventing you from experiencing closeness with those you love. Seek help if you need it. It will open the door to the love you really want.

THE POWER TO MAKE LOVE LAST

Is it possible for love to last for decades? There are couples who seem to stay romantically interested in one another throughout their married life. What's their secret?

Research by Bianca Acevedo and Arthur Aron, who are part of Helen Fisher's team, used fMRI scans to study the brains of happy couples in stable relationships for an average length of 21.4 years. The couples' brain activity was measured both while viewing facial images of their partner and while viewing images of a familiar acquaintance and a close friend. They found that greater satisfaction in marriage was related to activation of several brain areas specifically while viewing their partner. These included areas involved with reward and motivation, empathy, stress control, and the regulation of emotion. Greater marital satisfaction also was correlated with the area of the brain that regulates mood. Altogether, it's clear that couples with better relationships have brains associated with greater health and well-being. What is the direction of causation? We don't know from this research, but it is clear that relationships can be soothing or they can make you crazy.

Over my years working with patients, I've seen a variety of relationship types. I can also draw from my own personal experience—and the experiences of my friends and family—to know that love that lasts is the result of partners embedding themselves in each other's brains in a positive way. Memory circuits and pleasure get all wound up together so that the other person becomes integral to the very structure of your brain, and you become part of the structure of his.

Embedding yourself in your partner's brain is not hard to do. It does require motivation, dedication, and a little knowledge. I've come up with a list of twelve things you can do to make a lasting impression on the one you love and keep that love alive and growing. These are powerful actions. Don't use them unless you're serious about your relationship and intend to commit yourself to it.

Take Your Partner's Breath Away—Do something amazingly thoughtful and out of the ordinary. And let there be an element of surprise to it. A loving note tucked into a pocket. A special dinner on an otherwise ordinary night. A playlist made up with his favorite songs. These thoughtful acts will embed you in his memory.

Do Something Special on a Regular Basis—Call him every day to touch base and get his nervous system used to hearing your voice. Make his favorite meal once a week. Once he begins to expect these things, you will always be close to his awareness. Also, do something special intermittently. Random reinforcement is the most powerful form of conditioning. Plan romantic evenings on a random schedule so that he doesn't know when they'll happen but will always have a feeling of excited anticipation.

Engage in Lots of Eye Gazing—New couples seem to do this naturally, but don't drop this strong bonding behavior just because the relationship has progressed. This is one way to keep the romance alive and is especially powerful when making love.

Learn What Pleases Your Partner Sexually—Make it clear that his pleasure is your pleasure, and you want to discover everything about what turns him on. He'll be happy to have you experiment on him. Not only will you get more adept at pleasing him, but he will see that you are willing to make a special effort just for him.

Teach Your Partner What You Like—For most partners, pleasing you makes him feel good about himself. And research shows that the sexual pleasure of one partner increases the pleasure of the other partner. Dr. Irwin Goldstein cites evidence that when men take an impotence drug (Levitra), their partners have better sex because their bodies work better, with better lubrication and more intense orgasms. We sense our partner's level of arousal and are turned on by it. So by getting him to do what you want, he will sense your greater arousal, and he will be more aroused as well.

Boost Lasting Love with Sexual Novelty—When things get humdrum and routine, there is not going to be as much of a hormonal/neurotransmitter reaction, and arousal is lessened. A little novelty increases anticipation, more hormones are secreted, and more thrilling sex is the result. Keep this up throughout your relationship and the temptation to stray will be reduced.

Do Something a Little Edgy—If you get your partner's heart rate up, he may associate the feeling of excitement with you and he may develop more powerful feelings for you. Going on a roller-coaster ride, taking a balloon trip, shooting the rapids—anything with a touch of danger to it—can make him fall more deeply in love with you. No head injuries, of course.

Use Every Sense—Your partner has five senses. You can embed yourself in each one of them. For vision, wear sexy clothing that you know he likes, add the soft glow of firelight during your dates, and put a picture of the two of you on his desk. For sound, speak in a pleasing tone, and use music you know he likes. For touch, find out what pleases him when you're intimate. But even when you're just spending time together, touch him while you're talking, brush your hand on his arm as you walk by him, give him affectionate kisses. For taste, make sure your mouth tastes good when you kiss him. And smell is extremely important as it is linked to the most primitive part of his brain. Find out what smells he likes—and, more important, what he doesn't like. Whether he likes a certain perfume on you, or he prefers your natural scent, find out what smell drives him crazy, in a good way. That's what you want to wear.

Do Something Great for Someone Your Partner Loves—If you show kindness and love for someone he loves, you will earn major points. When you enter a relationship, you also enter a relationship with all his family and friends. He wants you to enhance the lives of those he loves. So show him that the people who are important to him are important to you. This includes children from a previous marriage, parents, friends, employees and employers, and pets. Your acts of kindness toward them are a powerful bonding technique that appeals to his limbic brain and embeds you deeply in his consciousness.

Summarize and Immortalize Loving Moments—Don't be afraid to give voice to your love. Tell him how you feel. Write a loving note or a poem. Lovers have been doing this from the beginning of time because it works.

Learn from Parrots—Barbara Wilson is a neurologist who keeps and trains parrots. She says they have taught her important lessons about relationships that many humans could benefit from: Share your food with the one you love, groom each other, sing constantly, build nests together, and repeat each other's words and actions. The repetition validates the other person and attests to your interest in one another. It's a powerful way of saying, "We're in this together. I recognize you, you're important to me. We're one."

Boost the Chemicals of Love—There are many brain chemicals that go into the feeling of love and attachment. Here is information on what you can do to enhance two of these chemicals. Oxytocin is known as the bonding, trust, and cuddle hormone. It works to increase our sense of connection and closeness to others. Oxytocin is enhanced by watching romantic movies together, holding hands, cuddling, and long, loving eye contact. Women usually have more oxytocin than men, but according to one study, a man's level of oxytocin goes up 500 percent after making love. Withholding sex or being too busy to make love pushes couples apart. Work to stay close. It is good for your attachment to each other. There is even a company now that makes an oxytocin spray to enhance love. I may have to get some to help me at home for the times I say stupid things and get myself into trouble. There is another love chemical called phenylethylamine, or PEA, which works deep in the brain to alert you that something fun is about to happen. Dark chocolate increases PEA, as do almonds and cheese. Cheese actually contains more PEA than chocolate. Hmmm. Has anyone besides me ever wondered why French restaurants have cheese on the dessert menu? Now you know. You are more likely to get "dessert" when you get home if you have cheese. Another sure way to boost the attachment chemicals in your brain is to focus on what you love most about your partner. If you're like most people, you have "the list" of the things you love about your partner and the things that irritate you. Where you focus your attention determines how you feel. If you focus on the things that bother you—say, that he is a slob—you will definitely feel bothered. If you focus most on what you love, such as he is one of the kindest people you have ever met, then you are so much more likely to feel loving toward him. Make of list of seven things that you are grateful for about your partner, and then meditate on just one of them a day. You will notice a positive difference in your relationship in less than a week.

The secret to being a great lover is to know the brain tendencies of your partner and then match your behavior to fit his or her brain.

There is not one "loving" strategy that works for everyone. Why? We all have different brains. Some of us are extroverts; some of us are introverts. Some of us have low activity in the front part of our brains, which makes us excitement seeking. So we are likely to love scary movies, motorcycles, a good argument, and need novelty in the bedroom. Others of us have too much activity in the front part of our brain, which makes us seek predictability. So we are likely to hate scary movies, hate motorcycles, hate a good argument, and hate novelty in the bedroom.

Knowing your partner's brain is essential! For example, if your partner has an "anxious" brain, likely he needs reassurance, a warm bath, soft music, and a foot rub in order to relax into being intimate. If your partner has an obsessive brain, you will get more love by being predictable, making sex his idea, playing soothing music, and watching what you say, because he never lets go of hurts.

Different brains need different strategies. Even the time of a woman's cycle matters, as your brain changes. At some times in your cycle, you might want your partner to be assertive and just take you; at other times, if your mate tries the same move, you will hit him upside his head.

Unfortunately, most people have no clue about the brain, so when they struggle in a relationship, they just think that they have fallen out of love and start looking for a new partner.

Most females want love and have built-in mechanisms for lasting, loving relationships. With a healthy brain and healthy hormones, you feel happier and sexier, and you can act in a consistent loving way that will attract more love into your life. You have the power to create amazing connections. And the rules and suggestions in this chapter can help you make the most of this inborn ability.

ASK FOR WHAT YOU WANT

Are you embarrassed to ask your partner for what you want? Try this exercise by filling in the blank for each item. Have your partner do it too. Then practice on each other. You can't read each other's minds. You have to learn to ask.

I like it when you _____ my hair.

I like it when you _____ my ears.

I like it when you _____ my eyes.

I like it when you _____ my nose.

I like it when you _____ my neck.

I like it when you _____ my upper back.

I like it when you _____ my lower back.

I like it when you _____ my breast/chest.

I like it when you _____ my belly.

I like it when you _____ my genitals.

I like it when you _____ my butt.

I like it when you _____ my thighs.

I like it when you _____ my lower legs.

I like it when you _____ my feet.

GRIEF AND TOUCH

Angela and Jose are one of my favorite couples. I initially saw them several years ago as part of a show on *Dr. Phil* about compulsive cheaters. Jose had serious problems, but through our work together he has made remarkable progress and has been sober for over three years. Two and a half years into treatment, Jose's father died suddenly. Like most people, he went through a period of grief. He was becoming more short-tempered and withdrawn. Angela was incredibly supportive. Over time, however, she didn't know whether to get irritated with him or to soothe him. She did not want to encourage his bad behavior, and she asked for my help.

When we lose people we love, our limbic or bonding centers tend to become overactive, making us more vulnerable to depression. As mentioned earlier, men tend to express depression as anger and social withdrawal, rather than sadness. My advice to Angela was that Jose needed more tenderness and touching and lovemaking. Oxytocin, the hormone of bonding, is less active in men, but it goes up 500 percent after he has an orgasm. There is research from my colleague Dr. K. Paul Stoller, who has had very good success using intranasal oxytocin to help with grief. He discovered it in himself, after experiencing suffocating grief after losing Galen, his sixteen-year-old son, in a train accident. I suggested Angela try touch and lovemaking to naturally boost oxytocin. If that didn't work, we were going to try intranasal oxytocin. The touch worked, and Angela and Jose's relationship continues to grow and strengthen.

Hour 10 Exercise—Be the Director of Your Pleasure

1. One-hour practice session with your partner, if you have one who is cooperative, or with a masseuse: The goal of this exercise is to learn about your body, to be curious about what you like and don't like. Make this an hour of uninterrupted time. Do not bring any expectations or pressure to the session, just your curiosity.

Directions with a love partner: Start with a brief general massage, head to feet, front and back; include all the areas you wish. Set a timer to massage each area for thirty seconds. Pick out the massage oil with a scent you love. Rate each area on a scale of 1 to 10, with 10 being the most pleasurable feeling. Recommended areas lying facedown: scalp, neck, shoulders, upper back, lower back, buttocks, back of upper legs, back of knees, back of lower legs, feet. Lying faceup: face, shoulders, arms (including inside of elbows and wrists), hands, breasts, belly, genitals (do not just tell him to stop here), inside of thighs, upper legs, lower legs, feet. Have your partner record your ratings for each area; that way he will know which areas you like the best. During this exercise, get out of your head and focus on the sensations in your body to learn what you like the most.

Directions with a masseuse: Follow the same procedure but do not include breasts or genitals. Have your masseuse record your ratings for each area; that way you will be able to communicate with your partner the areas you like the best. Again, during this exercise, get out of your head and focus on the sensations in your body to learn what you like the most.

BONUS EXERCISES:

What Turns You on the Most?

Do these brain exercises to discover your pleasure buttons:

> Ask your partner to use warming gel during a foot rub.
> Have your partner kiss you on both left and right side of your
> neck to see if you experience this sensation differently on
> either side.
> Try up to ten scents for ten seconds each. Scents you might
> try are baby powder, vanilla, cinnamon, orange, roses,
> musk, peppermint, jasmine, cucumbers, licorice

Practice Makes Perfect

Set up practice sessions with your partner. Tell him what you want. Tell him again until he gets it right.

Use Your Imagination

See how aroused you can get without being touched. Focus on different body parts—a finger, a toe, a nipple, or your clitoris. Imagine them being fondled and see which areas make your brain respond the most.

11

GET YOUR BRAIN READY FOR BABIES AND CARING FOR THEIR BRAINS ONCE THEY'RE HERE

PREPARE FOR PREGNANCY AND UNLEASH THE POWER OF YOUR DAUGHTERS' BRAINS

Getting your brain and body ready for babies and caring for their brains in the best possible way is the eleventh step to unleashing the power of the female brain.

When you are a mother, you are never really alone in your thoughts. A mother always has to think twice, once for herself and once for her child.

—SOPHIA LOREN

If you get your brain healthy, you are much more likely to encourage those you love to get healthy as well. Nowhere is this more true than when considering having and raising children. The information in this chapter will help you take control of the most important aspect of your pregnancy, which is your own health (especially your brain health), and the health of your baby.

GETTING READY FOR PREGNANCY

To give your baby the best start possible, you want to create a good environment within your body for it to grow in. You should begin working on this as early as possible. As soon as you decide you're going to try to become pregnant, begin following the brain-healthy plan you're learning here.

Begin a Healthy Diet Before You Become Pregnant—Having healthy babies requires eating a healthy diet. And a good diet needs to start before conception for the most benefit. Studies show that mothers who have poor diets prior to conception are more likely to have babies who have reduced birth weight and are at greater risk for developing obesity and type 2 diabetes. So if you're thinking of becoming pregnant, now is the time to start watching what you eat. That means lots of lean protein, good fresh fruits and vegetables, whole grains, and not a lot of sugar and processed food. Drink lots of pure water.

Take Supplements—Don't forget your supplements, including a good multivitamin and 400–800 µg of folate. Folate is a form of B vitamin that is essential to help prevent neural tube birth defects in developing babies. Dutch researchers report that the risk of emotional problems in children was significantly less when their mothers had adequate levels of folate. It's advisable to start taking it before you become pregnant and to continue taking it all through your pregnancy and while nursing. Beef liver, lentils, spinach, asparagus, avocados, green peas, broccoli, and papaya are good food sources of folate. I recommend that my patients also take a high-quality multivitamin to make sure they are getting the folate and other needed nutrients.

Quit Smoking—There is evidence that women who smoke not only have less chance of becoming pregnant, but they are at increased risk of having an ectopic pregnancy, in which the fertilized egg implants itself in a fallopian tube or elsewhere outside the uterus.

Engage the Help of Your Own Health Team—Have a checkup with your doctor early on to make sure there are no obvious problems. It a good idea to do this early, while you're still thinking about getting pregnant. Have your doctor do a test to check if you've ever had German measles (rubella), which can cause serious birth defects if you become infected while pregnant. If you haven't, and you're not yet pregnant, your doctor may suggest you get vaccinated against the disease. Also, gum disease can cause systemwide inflammation, so get your teeth cleaned and floss regularly.

It really isn't hard. The more you can do before you get pregnant to get fit and healthy, the more you'll be helping your baby get a good start in life.

DEALING WITH INFERTILITY

Obviously, there are many causes of infertility, including infections, trauma, ill health, low hormone levels, allergies, and many other possibilities. One of the most common causes of infertility is stress. Being unhappy, frequently upset, tense, or angry can clamp down on your fallopian tubes making it harder to conceive. Scientific evidence shows that chronic stress causes hormonal changes that disrupt reproductive function.

The same way that stress prematurely ages your body and skin, it also speeds up the aging process of your reproductive system. For women, it is harder to conceive as age advances, whether the aging is natural or stress-induced. Women aren't the only ones who suffer from infertility owing to stress. Researchers in India have found that emotional stress damages sperm cells. In addition to causing problems for natural conception, elevated stress levels also impact the success of fertility treatments, such as in vitro fertilization (IVF). Fertility treatments by themselves are universally enormously stressful!

A study published in *Human Reproduction* investigated the effects of stressful life events on IVF treatment. The researchers asked 809 women to complete a questionnaire about stressful and negative life events during the twelve months prior to undergoing fertility treatment. Women who became pregnant following treatment reported fewer stressful events than women who didn't conceive. The researchers concluded that stress may reduce the chances of a successful outcome following IVF treatment.

There's a commentary I love in the same journal from a psychologist on the faculty at UNED University in Madrid, Spain. He is convinced that stress is to blame for many cases of infertility and suggests that stress reduction should be the first course of treatment for infertility rather than expensive and invasive treatments, such as IVF. It makes sense to me: Stress reduction poses no side effects and doesn't involve any of the ethical or religious quandaries that come with some fertility treatments.

PREGNANCY

A ROLLER-COASTER RIDE OF HORMONES

Creating a baby is one of life's greatest miracles, and it takes a major revamping of your hormone balance to accomplish it. During pregnancy, and in the period following delivery, we see the largest fluctuation in hormones that a woman will ever experience in her life. A number of different hormones play major roles in the transformation and understanding what's happening to your body will help you cope with the changes.

Estrogen and progesterone are two of the most important hormones during pregnancy, and they are both produced in abundance during this time. However, the first hormone that comes into play is human chorionic gonadotropin (hCG), which is only released early in pregnancy and is not present at any other time in a woman's life. It is hCG that stimulates the ovaries to start producing greater quantities of estrogen and progesterone, and it is the presence of hCG that is picked up on by those home pregnancy tests.

As the pregnancy progresses, the placenta itself starts producing copious amounts of estrogen and progesterone, and at that point the quantity of hCG diminishes as it is no longer needed. Estrogen prepares the womb to receive the fertilized egg and readies the breasts for nursing. It also regulates the production of progesterone.

Progesterone builds the wall of the womb so that it can support the placenta. It also helps reduce randomly occurring contractions. In both these ways, it helps keep the womb from spontaneously aborting the fetus.

The pituitary gland produces the hormone prolactin, which is essential for milk production and nursing. As with much of the hormone system, it is the balance among different hormones that is essential for the harmonious execution of the body's functions. Estrogen and progesterone prevent prolactin from bringing about the production of milk prior to birth. After birth, estrogen and progesterone levels drop dramatically, which clears the way for prolactin to initiate milk production.

Oxytocin is a hormone that serves a number of important functions. It is heavily involved in labor by directing contractions. In fact, oxytocin is the drug that doctors use to artificially induce labor. But the hormone is also related to pleasurable feelings. Sometimes referred to as the cuddle chemical, it appears to be the hormone that underlies social bonding in general and is an important factor in a mother's bonding to her infant. The hormone, which is released in the brain during sexual arousal and orgasm, is also released when an infant nurses, building a bond of trust and pleasure between mother and baby. Researchers at Israel's Bar-Ilan University have found that greater amounts of oxytocin in the blood of pregnant women predicted stronger bonding between mothers and babies after birth as measured by gazing, touching, and vocalizing.

THE MOMMY BRAIN: DOES IT EXIST?
AND IS IT A MINUS OR A PLUS?

I knew a woman who only had two fender benders in her life. And both of them took place while she was pregnant with each of her two children. Her take on the situation was "I just can't drive when I'm pregnant."

Many women who are pregnant claim that they feel like there are lots of things happening to their brains that they don't understand. Their memories get foggy so it's hard to carry on a conversation or remember whether or not they put the baking powder into the cake batter.

Some researchers pooh-pooh the idea of a "mommy brain," but many other researchers, and women around the globe, claim that it's as real a phenomenon in pregnancy as a swelling belly. In fact, after reviewing the research, the American Psychological Association has concluded that 50–80 percent of women report decreased concentration and memory during pregnancy. But the paradoxical conclusion that some researchers are coming to is that some of these "symptoms" may actually be signs of changes in the brain that may end up making the woman smarter and better equipped to keep her child healthy and safe. The flood of reproductive hormones may actually prepare the brain for the demands of being a mother, making her a more sensitive and effective caretaker who is less disturbed by stress and more attuned to the needs of her infant. Psychologist Laura M. Glynn surmises this is why mothers are easily aroused when their babies stir, whereas their fathers stay blissfully asleep.

Glynn also reports that when the fetus moves in the womb, it raises the mother's heart rate and skin conductivity, which are signs of an emotional response. This may ready the mother to bond to her baby even before it's born. Fetal cells enter the mother's bloodstream through the placenta. "It's exciting to think about whether those cells are attracted to certain regions in the brain," Glynn says, which would mean the fetus is influencing the changing brain of its mother, preparing her to love it.

One surprising finding from fMRI scans is that a woman's brain may physically shrink during the third trimester of pregnancy. Anesthesiologist Anita Holdcroft has found that pregnant women's brains shrink an average of 3–5 percent. However, there is more here than first meets the eye. Dr. Louann Brizendine explains that the shrinkage does not seem to be the result of a loss of brain cells. Instead, it is due to changes in cellular metabolism. The shrinkage is a sign of brain circuits that are being restructured in preparation for their being changed from "one-lane highways" into "superhighways." And as research has continued to show, the brain does not shrink uniformly. Some very significant areas of the brain grow larger.

Don't worry: A few weeks postpartum, the brain starts getting bigger again and is usually returned to its normal size within six months. So it's bigger again, and better, because its improved circuitry is maintained. In animal studies, mother rats are better, more efficient learners who are less fearful and are therefore better providers for their families compared to females who have not borne a litter.

Researcher Craig Kinsley reported in 2011 that his mother subjects were more resistant to stress and had enhanced memory and cognition. Kinsley explains that the maternal brain undergoes a revolutionary change. At first it feels like a disorganized construction zone, which may account for the fuzzy thinking and other symptoms of the mommy brain. However, once the infant is born and the neuronal changes start taking hold and become organized, the result is a better brain that is more efficient and focused and that has been transformed from a self-centered organism to an other-focused caregiver.

Here's one example of an important change: Early in pregnancy, a woman's olfactory system changes, making her more aware of odors. It is believed that this makes her more sensitive to the smell of food that may be bad for her and the child growing inside her, and it is a critical mechanism for survival. Interestingly, that same change in her sense of smell makes her actually like the smells given off by her baby, including the smell of baby poop. It's all part of the bonding process that is guided by a number of neurological changes occurring in her brain.

Kinsley points out that the bonding process, all of which is designed to improve the survivability of the next generation, leads to other positive changes in the mother, including improvements in spatial memory and enhanced learning ability. And, according to the results of animal studies, these changes are essentially permanent, lasting well into old age.

So the finding is that the brain appears to shrink as it "rewires," but at the same time very important areas of the maternal brain grow. And these areas are directly related to increasing the mother's ability to take care of her babies. According to the American Psychological Association review of the literature, the main changes seem to involve increased size of the midbrain.

In research with humans, Pilyoung Kim, now at the National Institutes of Mental Health in Bethesda, Maryland, scanned the brains of new mothers a few weeks after giving birth and then again three to four months later. Her findings were consistent with earlier findings from animal studies: There were size increases in the hypothalamus, PFC, and amygdala. According to Kim, these areas of the brain are the seat of motivation and reward. She concluded that size increases in these areas are important for motivating the mother to care for her infant and make her feel rewarded by her interactions with her baby, especially by eye contact and smiles. In fact, the mothers who had the largest increases in the size of these areas were also the most enthusiastic about rating their babies as special, beautiful, ideal, and perfect. These areas of the brain are also critical for planning and foresight. They help the mother both anticipate her baby's needs and make the plans that are necessary to take care of them. This is the basis of "maternal instinct" with its love, fascination, worry, and need to protect. It's what helps her plan visits to the pediatrician in the middle of her busy workweek, sit in the waiting room and carefully watch anyone who approaches, prepare her list of questions to ask the doctor, and at the right time, dip into her tote bag filled with snacks and toys.

But if this is so, why the brain fog during pregnancy and postpartum? Some speculate it's just due to lack of sleep. But Kim, herself a new mother, has another idea, and she thinks it has to do with changing priorities. "We are clearly showing that mothers have better memories about things related to their infants. There are a lot of things going on, and mothers might feel forgetful about things that are not related to their infants. It's just dependent on what is really important for us to remember at the time."

A thorough review of available research was compiled by Katherine Ellison and presented in her book *The Mommy Brain: How Motherhood Makes Us Smarter*. As a Pulitzer Prize–winning reporter, she turned her skill for ferreting out information on the topic after noticing changes in herself as the result of her own two pregnancies. Ellison concludes, "The brain changes when you become a mother. It becomes more efficient, perceptive, motivated and empathetic—all useful skills in the workplace. Rather than a deficiency, as our culture emphasizes, it's actually an asset."

So, it appears there really is a mommy brain, but rather than being a problem, it may actually be a tremendous asset to a new mother. The transformation in a woman's brain may be designed to prepare her to be a better, calmer, more efficient mother, and the changes may benefit her for her entire life. Apparently a little fogginess may be the prelude to a new level of focus and intelligent action. There are many sacrifices in motherhood, but the entire process also contributes significant rewards to the mother's brain.

A HEALTHY PREGNANCY: WHAT TO DO

For thirty years, I've been talking about what all of us need to do to have a healthy brain. And, of course, what's good for the brain is good for the body. When you're pregnant, what's good for your brain and your body is also what's good for the little brain and body that are growing inside of you. Diligently follow the program in this book.

> **Exercise**—In the old days, pregnant women were treated as though they had some kind of illness. They were often advised that exercise was not a good idea, and back in fifties and sixties, exercise wasn't high on anyone's list of things to do anyway.
>
> Today many women exercise like crazy, and they're not about to give that up when they get pregnant. They're highly motivated to stay in shape. They think they'll have an easier time of pregnancy and the birth process itself if they stay active and fit. And research backs them up. Studies out of the Polytechnic Institute of Madrid show that low-level physical exercise throughout pregnancy has beneficial effects on the health of both mother and baby. They also found that exercise helped reduce some of the effects of the tendency of heavier mothers to give birth to heavier babies. Babies who are born with excessive weight face greater complications at birth and are more at risk of developing illnesses as adults, such as diabetes and some cancers. In the study, overweight mothers who were sedentary tended to give birth to heavier newborns. However, overweight mothers who exercised during pregnancy did not give birth to heavier babies.
>
> Exercise can help your body weather some of the changes it is going through. For example, it can help you maintain good posture, which can reduce backaches and other discomforts. It also reduces stress, and it builds your stamina to help you better get through labor and delivery. And some studies show that women who exercise are less likely to

get gestational diabetes, a temporary form of diabetes that develops in some women during pregnancy.

If you've had an exercise plan prior to becoming pregnant, you can modify it as needed to make sure you don't put a strain on you or your baby. If you become exhausted or breathless you may be compromising the supply of oxygen to your baby, so cut back. Don't let your heart rate get above 140 beats per minute or it may put your baby in distress. If you have not been exercising but want to begin, start slowly and work your way up. I like my patients to walk like they're late for forty-five minutes four times a week. Keep yourself hydrated and don't exercise if it's too hot. Don't engage in contact sports, and don't run on rough terrain or do anything that might make you fall. Use weights to tone, but don't lift anything heavy over your head. Basically, use common sense so that your exercise keeps you in shape without doing any potential harm to you or your baby.

There are certain medical conditions that may make it inadvisable to exercise while pregnant, so do check with your doctor. But if he or she says it's okay, exercising can bring many benefits.

And when it comes to one very special kind of exercise, a review of the literature shows that sexual activity during pregnancy does not harm the fetus, provided there are no risk factors involved, such as sexually transmitted diseases. Some research indicates that one of the benefits of sex, especially during the late stages of pregnancy, is that it seems to ward off early delivery. And a full-term baby has the best chance for a healthy delivery and a great start in life.

WHAT TO AVOID

Don't Ignore Your Weight—It is very important to maintain an optimal weight during pregnancy, and that means not allowing yourself to put on too many pounds. You know all the health problems associated with obesity for yourself. But did you know that you can pass all those problems along to your unborn child? Recent research indicates that overweight mothers are more likely to have children who are born overweight and who are more likely to be obese in adulthood. Obese mothers are also more likely to have children who suffer with ADHD in childhood. So try to follow the healthy guidelines for eating we just looked at, and help your child enter the world at a healthy weight.

Don't Smoke—When you smoke, not only are you putting poison in your body that gets carried through to the baby inside you, but you are cutting back on the fetus's supply of oxygen. The results can be devastating. In one recent study that appeared in the *British Journal of Psychiatry*, women who smoked while pregnant had children who were at greater risk of exhibiting psychotic tendencies as teenagers. In another study based on animal research, smoking during pregnancy produced offspring with faulty production of myelin, the fatty sheath that insulates brain connections. Without healthy myelin, impulses are not transmitted properly. The researchers concluded that this may explain the finding that mothers who smoke are more likely to have children who develop ADHD, autism, tendencies to drug abuse, and a host of psychiatric disorders.

Mothers who smoke also have more complications during pregnancy and may deliver preterm. Their babies often show low birth weight, and when they grow up they are more likely to show physical symptoms like asthma, sudden infant death syndrome, colic, and respiratory infections.

Smoking is a terrible thing to do to yourself and your baby.

Hold the Alcohol—Just as you stop smoking for your baby, you should also abstain from alcohol. There is evidence that abusing alcohol during pregnancy can lead to birth defects and fetal alcohol syndrome. It is also associated with conduct problems in childhood. But does that mean cutting out alcohol altogether? Some doctors say yes, that you should cut it out completely while you're pregnant. I agree. It is not giving you or the baby any benefit.

Don't Do Drugs—As with cigarettes and alcohol, anything you do, your baby does as well. If you are on prescription drugs, discuss your pregnancy with your doctor to see if any dosage changes are warranted. And if you are using recreational drugs, please stop. If you don't, your baby could pay the price for the rest of her life.

And what about caffeine? There is evidence that too much caffeine during pregnancy can lead to some birth defects, preterm delivery (and in some studies, but not all, miscarriages), and low birth rate. Do you know how your heart races when you have too much caffeine? Well, your baby's heart races as well. Some doctors say you should cut it out altogether while pregnant (and that includes the hidden caffeine in sodas, chocolate, and Excedrin). Some doctors say that under 150 mg caffeine a day is okay (about one and a half cups of coffee). A cup of green tea can be very satisfying, at just 40 mg. But to be on the safe side, cut out the caffeine altogether. It's a small sacrifice that could mean a lot for your baby's health.

Watch Cell Phone Use—For years some scientists have warned that the radiation emitted by cell phones can damage the brain. But more research has been needed. Now research is under way, and recent studies on mice at the Yale School of Medicine provides the first experimental evidence that exposing fetuses to cell phone radiation does in fact affect their behavior as adults. The researchers found that compared to a control group, mice that were exposed to cell phone radiation in utero suffered from hyperactivity and demonstrated problems with memory. The researchers said that studies with humans were necessary before drawing any final conclusions; however they said it may be advisable to limit fetal exposure to this form of radiation.

Let Your Partner Clean the Kitty Litter Box—A common parasite, *Toxoplasma gondii,* can lurk in the cat litter box. It is spread through cat feces, undercooked meats, and unwashed vegetables, and it has been known to cause still births or brain damage if transmitted from the mother to the baby. In a recent international study of more than forty-five thousand women, being exposed to this parasite also made women more prone to suicide. Washing your hands when dealing with animal waste is always important to your health but even more so when considering getting pregnant.

I know this may sound like a lot to give up for the sake of your baby (except for giving up cleaning the kitty litter box, which should be easy), but it will be well worth it to have a healthy baby and a healthier you, who will be better able to take care your family and meet the many other challenges we all face every day.

THE EMOTIONAL CONNECTION: IT STARTS EARLIER THAN YOU THINK

Many women talk about the special bond they feel with their children. There's scientific evidence that not only backs it up but that also indicates the connection starts very early in the relationship.

Laura Glynn explains that just as the fetus influences the development of the mother's brain, the influence goes the other way as well. Intrauterine signals influence the developing brain structure of the fetus as well as cognitive function and physiological stress regulation that will affect the child throughout his or her life.

For example, research at the University of Pennsylvania School of Nursing indicates that violent behavior in adulthood partially may be a function of the environment a fetus experiences in the womb. Specifically, prenatal and postnatal exposure to toxic elements like tobacco smoke or lead and poor maternal nutrition are related to delinquent behavior in teenagers, which is further related to violence in adults. Additional risk factors are maternal depression and stress, birth complications, traumatic brain injury, and child abuse.

With regard to maternal depression, a longitudinal study conducted by researchers at Cardiff University, King's College London, and the University of Bristol provided evidence that a mother's depression prior to birth is linked to violence in her children. Women who are depressed while pregnant are four times more likely to have children who are violent at age sixteen. This held for both sons and daughters. Somehow the mother's depression is creating a chemical environment in her womb that predisposes her children to express violent behavior later in life.

When you are pregnant, lines of communication and influence are opened between you and your baby, and whatever is communicated can have untold consequences on that baby's further development. If you are having any emotional problems, or problems with any addictions, don't ignore them. Seek the help you need now, and you may alter for the better the course of your child's future life.

POSTPARTUM

DEPRESSION AND PSYCHOSIS

During pregnancy, a woman's body is stoked with hormones. Then comes the birth, which is accompanied with a sudden, major shift in her hormone balance. All that estrogen and progesterone fall off a cliff. That sharp reverse in itself would be enough to throw anyone into a tailspin. But add to that the disruption in sleep with a newborn to care for, the stress of perhaps not knowing what to do and concerns over not being a good enough mother (especially if this is a first child), and a completely new family dynamic, and the stage is set for a huge (negative) emotional response.

If the response is not too extreme and doesn't last too long, we call it the baby blues. This is so common that it may occur in 45–80 percent of women within the first ten days of giving birth. Symptoms include depression, spells of crying, broken sleep, disturbed appetite, and perhaps most distressing, lack of feeling for her baby. In most cases, these symptoms disappear as hormones come back into balance and conditions "normalize."

But sometimes the symptoms don't go away, and postpartum depression develops. It happens about 10 percent to 15 percent of the time. And it's even more prevalent among teenage mothers, up to 26–32 percent. When it occurs, it's very distressing to mother, baby, and the entire family network. Serious symptoms often appear about four weeks postpartum, although they can sometimes first appear even months later. One day everything seems to be fine, and then six months later the bottom falls out and the mother feels like she just can't handle everything anymore.

Even more serious is a very rare condition, postpartum psychosis, which occurs about once or twice in one thousand births. Here the symptoms are more extreme and can lead to suicide or infanticide.

There are a number of contributing factors to postpartum depression, although the exact cause has not been determined. To the degree that hormone imbalance may be involved, anything a woman can do to maintain a healthy lifestyle, with good nutrition, adequate sleep, and avoiding toxins, can help. Also, keeping stress at a minimum and having good support from family and friends can have a positive effect. Avoid isolation at this difficult time.

Seek professional help if your symptoms don't start to fade after two weeks but stay the same or get worse, if your symptoms interfere with your work and make it hard to care for yourself or your baby, and you have thoughts of harming yourself or your baby. Getting your thyroid (as well as your other important numbers) checked is essential. Counseling can help, as can exercise, simple supplements according to your brain type (see chapter 6), hormone therapy, or antidepressants for depression or antipsychotics for delusions or hallucinations. It is very important for you to be under the care of an experienced health care provider if these are issues for you or someone you care about.

It's important not to ignore the problem, because it not only affects you but your baby and husband as well. Children of mothers who have untreated postpartum depression can experience a disruption of emotional attachment and exhibit problems later in life. They often have difficulty with eating and sleeping, they can be hyperactive and have temper tantrums, and they can show delayed language development. And depression that is untreated can last up to a year or longer and even lead to chronic depression or later episodes of severe depression. So don't write off the condition as being "normal."

GENERATIONS OF HEALTHY BRAINS: UNLEASHING THE POWER OF YOUR CHILD'S BRAIN

Now that you've done everything you can to make sure that your brain is in the best condition for your own sake and the sake of your baby, it's time to think about the next generation and what you can do to keep your child's brain in good shape.

1. Take Good Care of Your Own Brain and Your Relationship with Your Baby's Father—Too many women ignore their own needs or their primary love relationship in favor of taking care of the children, but it is a mistake. Of course you need to take care of the children's basic needs, but if you neglect your own, your own unhappiness will leak through and affect their development.

2. Create an Enriched Environment Full of Attention, Eye Contact, Touching and Play—Just the right amount of stimulation helps the baby's brain develop. Singing, music, toys, and movement are all important to brain development.

3. Pass Along Your Healthy Eating Lifestyle—When it comes to eating behavior, children tend to eat the way their mothers do. In a study at Michigan State University, toddlers were less likely to eat a healthy amount of fruits and vegetables if their mothers did not. And we know that food preferences established in childhood persist through life. Anything that's good for you is good for your child. Eat a balanced diet with lean protein, plenty of fresh fruits and vegetables, moderate amounts of healthy fats (children need them to keep their brain in optimal shape), with a minimum of processed foods and sugar and little to no caffeine. Work together on planning meals and snacks that will nourish body and brain.

4. Start Healthy Habits Early—Since our daughter Chloe was two years old, she and I have been playing "Chloe's Game." This game is based on a very simple question: "Is this good for my brain or bad for it?" For example, if I said, "Avocado," she would say, "Two thumbs up!" If I said, "Chocolate cookies," she would respond, "Thumbs down. Too much sugar." If I said, "Boxing," she would say, "Two thumbs down. The brain is too soft to put it in a helmet and slam it up against other people." If I said, "Blueberries," she would question, "Are they organic? Blueberries hold more pesticides than any other fruit. But organic blueberries are great."

One day when Chloe was seven and we were in line for the Pirates of the Caribbean ride at Disneyland, she and I wrote a list of those things that were good and bad for the brain. We started by thinking of words, using the letters of the alphabet. It is a great exercise to do with children to get them thinking about their brains.

For example:

Good

Almond milk

Almonds

Anteaters (to eat the ANTs)

Apples

Apricots

Arithmetic

Avocados

Badminton

Bananas

Baseball

Basketball

Beans

Bell peppers

Berries

Bowling

Broccoli

Carrots

Cauliflower

Cinnamon

Cooperation

Creativity

Cucumbers

Cuddling

Dancing

Doodling

Drawing

Bad

Abuse

Alcohol

Anger

ANTs

Anxiety

Bad attitude

Bad behavior

Being too bossy

Boxing

Brain injuries

Bullying

Candy

Churros

Cookies

Cotton candy

Driving too fast

Drugs

 View Chloe's Entire List

5. Promote Brain-Healthy Exercise and Protect Them from Brain Injuries—The statistics are frightening. Did you know that every fifteen seconds, right here in the United States, someone experiences a traumatic brain injury? That's according to the Brain Injury Association of America. Brain trauma, even those that are considered mild, have been linked to aggressive behavior, depression, learning problems, panic attacks, and drug and alcohol abuse later in life. Up to 70 percent of injuries affect the PFC, the part of the brain concerned with planning, decision making, and impulse control. Damage to this part of the brain not only can lead to learning deficits, but it can also result in problems with controlling emotions and reading and responding appropriately to social signals.

Brain injuries come in many sizes. It's obvious that a trauma that leads to loss of consciousness is bad and requires immediate attention. But a series of small injuries can also add up to a major problem. Repetitive falls, head banging, or repetitive blows or concussions in football or soccer can be just as debilitating over time as one big blow.

It turns out that when it comes to the severity of symptoms following brain trauma, girls are at a disadvantage. In the most extreme cases of trauma in children under ten years of age, girls are more than four times as likely as boys to die from severe brain trauma. It's thought that higher levels of testosterone in boys protects their brains by building brain mass in the same way that it makes their muscles bigger and stronger. Estrogen in girls, however, makes them more susceptible to injury. Interestingly, whatever the cause of this difference, it reverses later in life. Among people in their fifties to seventies, women are twice as likely to survive serious brain trauma as men.

It's extremely important to protect developing brains. Of course children should wear helmets when riding bicycles, and they should not hang upside down on monkey bars placed above a concrete slab. But please also consider injuries that could take place during common sports. It isn't good for any child to engage in contact sports involving head butting or possible blows to the head. Football and soccer are not safe for anybody's brain, let alone a child's. This used to be primarily an issue for boys, but today girls are engaging more and more in these activities, and as we just saw, their brains are even more vulnerable than their brothers' and male classmates' are.

Flying soccer balls are a real menace. It is estimated that a ball that's been kicked hard can impact a player's head with a force of 175 pounds! Now think about your daughter's delicate little skull and the precious brain that's resting inside. Does that sound like a good idea to you? She's meeting that missile with her frontal lobes, and she needs those frontal lobes for the rest of her own life so that she can be a good mother to your granddaughters as the next generation comes along.

And even cheerleading, which used to be a fairly safe, fun activity, is becoming potentially very dangerous as it is being turned into an extreme sport. Now girls are "flyers" who are tossed up into the air, and if they don't stick the landing, there can be serious injury.

There are many healthy, enjoyable sports that will not compromise your daughter's brain health and her future. Tennis, Ping-Pong (my personal favorite), all forms of swimming, basketball, and volleyball, are all wonderful ways to exercise a growing body. And there are always ballet and other forms of dance. Encourage your daughter to have fun doing what's good for her.

6. Get Treatment for Any Emotional Issues or Learning Challenges Right Away—If you suspect your child has a behavioral, emotional, or learning issue, have it checked into. Small problems left untreated can turn into large problems. But early treatment can nip difficulties in the bud and change the entire course of your child's life. Sometimes all that's needed is a lifestyle change or the use of natural supplements. The sooner you get your child on a brain-healthy program, the better. A good place to start is by mentioning your concerns to your child's physician.

HELPING YOUR DAUGHTER THROUGH ADOLESCENCE: KEEPING HER SAFE UNTIL HER PFC KICKS IN!

Now that you've gotten your daughter safely through childhood, the next hurdle looms: adolescence. That's when your sweet little girl turns into a texting, tweeting, eye-rolling teenager who suddenly knows much more than you ever did and doesn't have the time or interest in any advice you may want to give her. However, without having a fully functioning PFC, the decisions she makes can be a little scary.

The PFC, the CEO of the brain that analyzes, plans, and controls impulses, is one of the last regions of the brain to fully develop. That means the girl who is learning to drive, who is going on dates, and who is being faced with all kinds of new situations and temptations, is not working with the full capacity of the part of her brain that can anticipate consequences, regulate intense emotions, and balance short-term gratification against long-term goals. That part of the brain doesn't fully mature until she reaches around twenty-five years of age. That allows a good ten years or so during which she has the means to take actions she may later regret.

And that's not good, because adolescents are especially vulnerable to permanent brain injury as a result of risky behavior.

Amphetamine Abuse—Information presented at the Society for Neuroscience indicates that amphetamine abuse during adolescence "permanently changes brain cells." According to research on animals, changes in electrical properties of cortical brain cells occurred after drug exposure during adolescence but not young adulthood. Other research shows that adult rats exposed to amphetamines in adolescence showed deficits in their working memory. It now appears that the change in cognitive behavior may be partially the result of changes to the function of neurons in the PFC as a result of amphetamines, which disrupt the normal process of brain development.

Cigarette Smoking—UCLA researchers have looked at brain function in adolescent smokers, focusing on the PFC. They found that the more a teen was addicted to nicotine, the less active the PFC. They concluded that smoking affects brain function, and the PFC is especially vulnerable because adolescence is a critical time for development of this brain region.

Marijuana—Researchers at the University of Cincinnati have concluded that the brains of teens who use marijuana work harder than the brains of their peers who do not use the drug. According Krista Medina, the lead researcher, "Chronic, heavy marijuana use during adolescence—a critical period of ongoing brain development—is associated with poorer performance on thinking tasks, including slower psychomotor speed and poorer complex attention, verbal memory and planning ability." Her findings also indicate that while there may be partial recovery of verbal memory functioning within three weeks of starting abstinence, there are long lasting effects as "complex attention skills continue to be affected." She also found that compared to boys, girls have a greater tendency to have cognitive problems, including poor executive function and a decreased ability to plan, make good decisions, and stay focused.

Eating Disorders—Another big problem girls are facing today is the growing level of obesity and eating disorders, both of which can interfere with proper brain function. Your relationship with your daughter is crucial in helping her develop good eating habits, healthy self-esteem, and a positive body image. A study reported in the *Archives of Pediatrics and Adolescent Medicine* found that the desire of teenage girls to maintain a good weight was partly based on how they perceived their mother's goal for them. That means if you instill in them the value to stay at a healthy weight, that will influence them positively. I think we can also conclude that if you have an overcritical view of your daughter's weight, it could lead to poor body image and perhaps even encourage the development of eating disorders. Be aware of the messages you are giving your daughter. You may not be aware of the messages you are presenting, but she will be aware on some level. Make sure your influence is for her good and yours.

Sleep Deprivation—According to the National Sleep Foundation, the average sleep requirement for a thirteen- to nineteen-year-old teenager is nine hours. How many teens even come close to that? I would wager not very many. But not getting enough sleep disrupts hormone regulation and can lead to putting on weight. It interferes with focus and willpower, reduces athletic performance, and is associated with depression and ADD; in other words, it creates havoc with everything important to a teenager's life. And sleep deprivation is rampant among teens. Sleep cycles change when kids reach their teen years. They are more apt to want to go to sleep later and wake up later. But school schedules that start early in the morning make it impossible for them to make up for the hours of sleep lost from texting and playing video games into the wee hours. Research with mice suggests that even short-term sleep restriction during adolescence can interfere with the balanced growth and depletion of brain synapses, which are the connections between nerve cells where communication occurs. The researchers surmise this can lead to long-term problems with the wiring of the brain. Adolescent girls may think that going to bed early "is for babies," a belief that can have lasting consequences.

Depression—Depression can hit anyone, but adolescent girls seem to be especially prone to it. They are twice as likely to experience bouts of depression compared to their male peers. Canadian researcher Nancy Galambos of the University of Alberta found that one in five teenage girls admit to undergoing periods of depression, as compared to one in ten boys. She goes on to say that depression is associated with anxiety, eating disorders, disruptive conduct, failure in school, and difficulty in relationships. Hormonal changes in girls may be a causal factor. Watch for signs of depression, like moodiness, isolation, self-harming behaviors like cutting or hair pulling, and seek help when behaviors begin to raise red flags.

Alcohol—Alcohol abuse by teens is an obvious problem when it leads to drunk driving and accidents. A recent report from the Mayo Clinic reveals that hospitalizations resulting from underage drinking have an estimated price tag of $755 million each year. Mayo Clinic addiction expert and psychiatrist Terry Schneekloth, M.D., says, "When teenagers drink, they tend to drink excessively, leading to many destructive consequences, including motor vehicle accidents, injuries, homicides and suicides."

Perhaps we associate this tendency more with boys more than girls, and in fact boys do make up 61 percent of alcohol-related hospitalizations of teens. But that means that 39 percent were girls, a significant amount. This is very troubling because not only do girls face the usual dangers associated with alcohol abuse, but they face another danger that they, and you, may not even be aware of: Adolescent girls and young women who drink alcohol have increased risk of benign (noncancerous) breast disease. This is not as benign as it sounds, as this is an increased risk factor for breast cancer later in life. And further research shows that the risk increases for adolescent girls from families with a history of breast cancer.

Risky Behavior in General—Researchers from the Netherlands have investigated the development of addictive behavior. Their conclusion? Addictive behavior has a greater likelihood of being initiated during adolescence than during any other period of life. It appears that the differential developmental trajectories of those brain regions specifically involved in motivation and self-control tend to make adolescents generally more prone to risk taking. And these tendencies are aggravated by the consequences of using drugs. Neuroimaging studies of adolescent brains show an imbalance between the impulse-controlling PFC and the deeper regions that are related to motivation. It is this imbalance during adolescence, when the PFC is not yet mature, that may be the cause of more risk-taking behavior at this time.

In related studies, the researchers looked at anticipation of reward in ten- to twelve-year-olds, fourteen- to fifteen-year-olds, and eighteen- to twenty-three-year olds. They found that of all the groups, the adolescents appeared to be hypersensitive to rewards. Everything just seems to promise so much more pleasure to them, possibly contributing to their greater risk-taking behavior.

So what's a mother to do? At a time when your daughter's brain is most vulnerable to negative influences that could interfere with proper development, she is also most tempted to engage in risk-taking behaviors that could cause lasting damage. How do you protect her?

First, your understanding of what's going on inside your daughter's head will help you in your dealings with her. You expect her to act like an adult, and she wants to be treated like an adult, but now you know she doesn't have the brain of an adult. So you are the one who has to be the adult. Instead of losing your cool and seeing her as trying to provoke you, keep your head and understand that she has a less mature perspective. Then give her the facts that can help her make better decisions. This is an excellent time to instill in her a little brain envy. Explain to her that there can be negative consequences to the things she now sees as fun and help her see the bigger picture, including the kind of future she really wants to have. Show her the brain scans in this book and on our website that clearly demonstrate the effect risky behaviors have on the brain. And engage her cooperation in a mother–daughter pact whereby the two of you work together to both have better brains. That means a better diet, exercising, and helping each other avoid harmful activities.

As each generation takes the responsibility of preparing for the next, the gift of brain health will be passed along, and all of us will benefit.

Hour 11 Exercise—Indulge in Special Time

I have taught parenting classes for many years. "Special Time" is one of the most effective exercises I have ever given to parents. It takes just twenty minutes for each child, but will make a huge difference in your relationship with your children. The exercise strengthens the parent–child bond.

Here it is: Spend twenty minutes a day with your child/teen doing something that he or she wants to do. During that time, issue no commands, ask no questions, and offer no directions. It is not a time to talk to her about her messy room, homework, or lack of respect. It is just a time to be together. The best time to start this is with young children, but I have also seen it be very powerful for older children and teenagers. Tell the children you miss them and just want to spend more time with them and that you want to make this a regular date, daily, if possible. Allow them to choose what you do together as long as it is safe, brain-healthy, and you can do it in twenty minutes. If you can do this every day, you will notice a significant boost in bonding within two weeks.

If you don't have children, do it with your partner. Bonding prolongs life and makes it worth living.

12

CHANGE YOUR FEMALE BRAIN, CHANGE THE WORLD

REALIZE THAT IT'S NOT ABOUT YOU— IT IS ABOUT GENERATIONS OF YOU

Creating a brain-healthy family and community is the twelfth
step to unleashing the power of the female brain.
Be the change you want to see in the world.

—MAHATMA GANDHI

While I was leaving church with my wife recently, a woman came up to us and said she had lost 45 pounds on the Daniel Plan, the health plan we helped to create at Saddleback Church. As she got healthy, her husband, who was 300 pounds at the beginning of our program, was also down 75 pounds. He did not start right away, but as he saw his wife's success, he decided to join her. She had told him that she was sorry he would not be around to enjoy a wonderful life with her. There was no nagging or belittling. She showed by example that a better life is possible if you do the right thing.

I hope you know from your own experience that you, as an individual woman, can change your own life and the lives of your friends and family. But let's take a minute to look at the bigger picture and get a more global perspective. Around the world, women are trying to do the same thing you are: Build a better life by changing themselves and the conditions around them. And when one woman unleashes the power of her brain, it's a huge stride forward for the betterment of all of us—male and female, young and old.

In their remarkable book *Half the Sky,* married journalists Nicholas Kristof and Sheryl WuDunn describe the heart-wrenching conditions of poverty and abuse under which women live around the world. They provide amazing stories of survival and transcendence in which brave, passionate women have turned tragedy to triumph to bring unimaginable healing change to themselves and their communities.

Leaders everywhere are realizing that the hope of the world lies in giving opportunity to women. As Kofi Annan, former secretary-general of the United Nations, said in his address to the "Women 2000" special session of the UN General Assembly, "Study after study has confirmed that there is no development strategy more beneficial to society as a whole—women and men alike—than one which involves women as central players."

In worldwide efforts to eliminate poverty, it has been found that helping women first to develop their own businesses creates a wave of prosperity that lifts the entire community. From microfinance loans to women through the Grameen Bank (founder Muhammad Yunus won the Nobel Peace Prize for his work), to the efforts of BRAC (the largest antipoverty organization in the world) to save lives and raise incomes of the poorest women, it's been proven again and again that women do not just benefit from the poverty-fighting efforts of others on their behalf, but they themselves become the most effective agents of the desired change.

And, in fact, if you look around the world you can see women leading efforts to bring about social changes that not only improve conditions for themselves, but also benefit their families and the larger community. They are calling for fairness in honoring water and land rights. They are pushing for improvements in education and health care. They are speaking up for better treatment of people who have no voice to speak for themselves. And they are working to bring about the resolution of conflict through better communication and understanding.

There's a growing acknowledgment by governments and aid workers that if you want to improve a community, you'd best start by giving more power and economic freedom to the women. When Kristof and WuDunn mentioned the politically incorrect opinion that women in Africa "typically work harder and handled money more wisely than men" to Festus Mogae, the enlightened former leader of Botswana, he agreed wholeheartedly: "You couldn't be more right. Women do work better. Banks were the first to see that and hired more women, and now everybody does. In homes too, women manage affairs better than men." It's widely accepted that when women are given more power, the lives of all the people improve.

It is critical that you recognize the power you have—not only to change yourself but those around you. Your female brain is compassionate and caring. Your intelligence is characterized by the ability to see the bigger picture and make connections. And whether you're looking to change the quality of life in the larger world around you or within your own home, you have the unique perspective and passion that can make you turn any situation into a better one. Given the right tools, you can be unstoppable.

THE POWER OF COMMUNITY

You can do remarkable things on your own. But you can be an even greater agent for change when your efforts are magnified by the power of community.

Dr. Linda Wagener, a leadership consultant from Marigold Associates says, "If I can only give people one piece of advice about how to make a change, I'll recommend that they surround themselves with people who embody that change." She goes on to give a number of specific reasons why being part of a community that supports change is so helpful. First, it provides a mirror to us, so we see ourselves more truly without underestimating or overestimating our strengths and weaknesses. We can use that information to make our actions more effective. Working with others also gives us the encouragement to go beyond what we think we can do. This is important when we're nervous about trying something new. Community also provides accountability to follow through on what we promise. We're more likely to visit the gym every day or take that brisk walk if we have a friend who is waiting for us to show up. And community gives us the support we need when we get discouraged and want to quit.

Many cultures are aware that change happens with the support of others. In her book *Join the Club: How Peer Pressure Can Transform the World*, Tina Rosenberg talks about the "social cure." She explains that usually when people try to bring about change, they do it by sharing information in an attempt to convince others. But the social cure takes a more direct approach. It changes behavior by helping people get what they care about most, which is the respect of their peers. Rosenberg believes that social pressure through a peer group—what she means by a club—is the best way to influence behavior. The peer group is so strong and persuasive, it can cause a woman to adopt a new identity as a member of the club. And she emulates the behavior of other club members: "I can be like my friend whose life has changed."

Possibly the most famous and successful of these "clubs" is Alcoholics Anonymous. Weight Watchers is another great example. Put someone with others who have the same goal, and together they form an entity that pressures each individual to meet the group goal.

Researchers give us some insight into why working in a group can be so effective. First, being part of a community helps relieve chronic stress. That removes a key factor in obesity, memory problems, cardiovascular and digestive issues, insulin dysregulation, and weakened immune system. On the positive side, being in a supportive group elevates stress-reducing hormones like oxytocin. That's why getting together with your friends for a chat where lots of bonding is going on can lead to a euphoric kind of peace.

Rosenberg believes that much of the dissatisfaction people have in life is due to feeling isolated. People are seeking community and connection. The social cure may involve a sacrifice of time for meetings, and a loss of privacy, but it solves important personal problems and adds meaning to people's lives. Getting others to join you in your endeavors is a great way to improve your chances of success.

Whether it's tackling personal health goals, trying to improve the environment, or bringing about social change, working with others first multiplies your efforts and, second, helps keep you on track. And women's brains are especially suited to effective action within a group setting. You have excellent communication skills, you easily make connections between ideas, you're great at multitasking, and you are empathic and compassionate. Also, friends can provide realistic, positive feedback when your own thoughts become negative, self-judgmental, and let's face it, a bit unreasonable.

As much as good company keeps you on track, bad company can derail you, so do be aware of the kind of company you keep. The power of social influence cuts both ways, and if you spend time with people who are unhappy, negative, or who engage in unhealthy habits, they can bring you down instead of raising you up.

There have now been a number of studies that show that unhealthy habits can be contagious. For example, research published in the *New England Journal of Medicine* found that one of the strongest associations in the spread of obesity was who you spend time with. This multigenerational heart study looked at data from over twelve thousand subjects over a thirty-year period. Subjects who had a friend who was obese had a 57 percent chance of also being obese. If the two individuals identified each other as being strong friends the figure shot up to 171 percent. And this relationship held even if the subjects didn't live in the same area. Sibling relationships also proved important. Having an obese sibling was related to a 40 percent increase in the chance of obesity.

Clearly, we influence each other for good, or for bad. Be aware of the influences around you. But also take this as a powerful motivator to be a good role model and a positive influence on the people with whom you interact. We know that when health-conscious friends improve their own health, their friends' health also improves. You can be the one who encourages others to do better by doing better yourself.

And the more you help others, the more you will help yourself. I like to think of it this way: *You have to give it away to keep it.*

I saw a great example of this one evening at an event in my own home. My wife runs a group through the Amen Clinics that helps women lose weight and get healthy. To celebrate the last class of the session, Tana was holding a party for the group members. They sounded like they were having so much fun, I couldn't resist joining in.

I got into a conversation with one of the woman who told me she had taken the class to learn how to deal with fibromyalgia and brain fog. Within two weeks of starting the program, the fibromyalgia symptoms were gone and her mind was much clearer. She had also dropped 11 pounds, which had been her goal. She said that she felt our program had changed her life.

I congratulated her on her progress and told her that to keep improving she had to give the program away by teaching others what she had learned. She replied that she had already begun. Her husband and children had started to eat better, and instead of sharing cookies with her co-workers, she was sharing information about healthy food. She had learned for herself that when you share your knowledge with others, you more firmly embed that wisdom into your daily life.

This is how you can be the agent for change. Reaching out to others so you can get healthy together helps both of you. And there are many benefits to your health, your well-being, the way you look and feel, and the quality of your relationships. It's a win-win for everyone—*and it all starts with you.*

A PRACTICAL APPLICATION: THE DANIEL PLAN

Being involved with the Daniel Plan at Saddleback Church has been one of the highlights of my life. The program was specifically designed to use the power of community to help individuals achieve healthier, more productive lives. The Daniel Plan is named after the biblical prophet who refused to eat the king's bad food. The fifty-two-week program has had remarkable success. One of the reasons it works so well is that we take advantage of a long-standing structure at Saddleback, where thousands of people meet each week in small groups. Few people can make major changes alone. Getting people into small groups enhances the commitment and learning of individuals by providing ongoing encouragement and emotional support. In fact, people are 50 percent more successful at weight loss and wellness improvement if they work in the context of a community rather than on their own.

The entire Daniel program is directed by Dee Eastman, a fitness and wellness expert with vast experience in small-group leadership. Dee stresses the power of community that develops in groups as members watch others they trust following the program, share information with one another, and engage in "water-cooler talk" that keeps group interests uppermost in members' minds. And when people have bad days, the group environment encourages members to pause and reflect without self-judgment and then ask for support to help bring balance into their lives.

Dee offers some great tips for making small groups succeed. You should keep these in mind if you're thinking of joining or creating your own support group. They can help make your efforts much more effective.

Be Authentic—The success of the group depends on the level of authenticity it encourages, and group members always follow the level of vulnerability and openness shown by the leader. In that regard, then, the speed of the leader is the speed of the team. Do not feel like you have to have it all together yourself to lead a group. Just being a woman who is open to growing and acting in a community setting is enough. You don't have to be the strongest in the group to lead. The focus should be on coming together in an open and honest place where there is a common desire to grow, change, and keep moving forward.

Have Some Accountability—Each group must decide what level of accountability members feel comfortable with, but there do need to be tangible goals that inspire members, and that all members are "behind" everyone achieving. Accountability can be implemented by giving reports at meetings, regularly checking in with one another, or any other system that works effectively.

Keep It Fresh—Don't get into a rut of going over the same material at every meeting. Vary the material studied, whether it's a new book, a DVD series, magazine articles, or anything else that's relevant, informative, and inspiring. Keep the material fresh and interesting so members will feel they're always getting something new and important, and their interest level is kept up. Variety is the spice of life when it comes to small groups!

Be Great Listeners—Group members should be great listeners for one another. They should seek to understand and come alongside one another; they should not try to solve the problems of people in the group. A comfortable, open atmosphere allows for openness and sharing. Feeling judged, or that others who think they know more are trying to fix you, is what closes people down.

Give Back—Your program should include ways of giving back to the church, culture, or community. Looking and giving outward balances the effort to grow inwardly. Sharing what has been learned extends the reach of the group's positive developments.

Draw Out Each Individual's Strengths—Dee says one of her favorite parts of the small group experience is seeing each individual's passion and calling revealed and then creating a platform where those gifts can be shared within the group and with the larger world. She creates opportunities for people to shine, perhaps by asking them to host a workshop or a food demonstration, appear in a video, write an article, and so on. She is always providing new leadership opportunities for others to serve within the group, to the benefit of the individual and the group. She works to foster these growth experiences and discourages competition. She says, "As women we can truly champion other women—draw out each other's strengths, provide opportunities for others to grow—so everyone wins and we operate as we were designed to live."

One of the most exciting outcomes of the Daniel Plan is seeing the group members spread what they've learned outside their small groups to their families and communities, thereby becoming a significant influence for healthy living. There is a tremendous domino effect for the positive. Dee gives an example of one group member, Chloe, who has lost an amazing 155 pounds. Not only has she become a new person, but she's sharing her new knowledge by writing on wellness and starting a healthy line of cupcakes. "And they are so delicious—go figure!" Dee adds.

YOU ALWAYS GET BETTER FASTER WHEN YOU ENGAGE THE FOUR CIRCLES

One of the problems with change is that it doesn't always last. You stick to your diet until the holidays roll around, and then you lose all control. You keep up with your exercise plan for a full month, and then you start skipping days and finally forget all about it.

You want more than a temporary change. You want change that lasts. And that requires change that radiates through your whole being and involves every part of you to become "locked in." For that kind of change to occur, it is critical that you engage each of the Four Circles talked about throughout the book (biology, psychology, social connections, and spiritual health).

Find a way to hook the change you want into each of those four aspects of your being, and it will be much more likely to be permanent. Do the same for the people you want to influence, and they will also see change that becomes ingrained into their nature.

DEVELOP GREAT COMMUNICATION SKILLS

To be an agent for change, you have to communicate effectively. Here are six ways to become a better communicator:

1. Assume the other person wants to communicate with you. Drop any negative attitudes on your part that may be setting you up for a bad outcome.

2. State what you want in a clear, positive way. Don't make demands that can be met with hostility. Don't be weak, which can lead to your being dismissed. Be firm, kind, and confident.

3. Decrease distractions and make sure you have each other's full attention.

4. Ask for feedback to make sure the other person understands you and that you understand the other person.

---

5. Be a good listener. Unless you both express what you want to say, there will be no communication, but there may be resentment and hard feelings.

6. Follow up on your communication. Even if you thought you reached an understanding, people forget, get distracted, or change their minds. If the outcome you want is important to you, follow up to see if the change you want is being implemented.

IT'S NOT JUST ABOUT YOU— IT'S ABOUT GENERATIONS OF YOU

Your behavior influences the expression of your genes and the health of subsequent generations. As Americans, we covet our freedom. We don't like anyone else telling us what to do, especially if it involves our own bad habits. But the unfortunate truth is that your behavior is not just about you. It is ultimately about generations of you. When Tana and I first figured this out, we became much more serious about our own behavior and what we did and did not allow in our home, and subsequently at the Amen Clinics.

A new field of genetics has grown up in the last twenty years called epigenetics. Epigenetic means "above or on top of the gene" and refers to the recent discovery that your habits and emotions can impact your biology so deeply that there are changes in the genes that are transmitted to the next several generations. It is these epigenetic "marks" that tell your genes to switch on or off, to express themselves loudly or softly. It is through epigenetics that immediate environmental factors like diet, stress, toxins, and prenatal nutrition can affect your genes that are passed to your offspring and beyond.

It is not just about you, it is about generations of you. For instance, a recent study has shown that boys who started smoking before puberty (say at age eleven or twelve) caused their sons to have significantly higher rates of obesity. This means that a dumb decision at age eleven can cause disastrous results for later generations. And obesity is just the beginning. Some researchers believe that epigenetics holds the key to understanding some cancers, forms of dementia, schizophrenia, autism, and diabetes.

In groundbreaking research, Dr. Lars Olov Bygren, a preventive-health specialist from Sweden studied the offspring of families who had experienced both feast and famine. Children and grandchildren of mothers who were malnourished had a higher incidence of heart disease. Counterintuitively, boys and girls who were born in times of feast (abundant food) produced children and grandchildren who lived significantly shorter lives. Eating too much, it seems, can be as bad on subsequent generations as eating too little. In these times of abundant food and epidemic overweight and obesity, this study should give all of us serious pause. What we eat can affect future generations. So you're not only what you eat but potentially what your mother and father and even grandparents ate too.

Another example of epigenetics is stress. When mothers-to-be are stressed they produce more of the hormone cortisol than they otherwise would. Some of the cortisol is transmitted to the baby through the placenta. The elevated stress hormones prematurely reset the baby's brain to be more sensitive or hyperresponsive to subsequent stressful events. For example, there is a very high incidence of depression in children of Holocaust survivors. Learning to manage your stress is important for you and your children and grandchildren.

Clearly, your behavior matters beyond yourself and is an important reason to get healthy *now*.

UNLEASH THE POWER THAT CAN
CHANGE YOUR WORLD

I am not a big believer in baby steps. I think for you to get healthy and stay that way you need to make a serious commitment. Tana, who is not only my wife but also my partner in helping people get well, says that to get really healthy people have to jump the canyon, which you cannot do in baby steps. It takes a leap to leave behind a toxic lifestyle.

Live your own best vision for yourself, and you can't help but better the lives of those you care about. As a woman, you bring special skills and talents to every task and every relationship. Unleash that power and there's no telling how far that positive influence can go.

Here are just three ways in which you can exert your amazing power of positive impact:

Be a Positive Role Model—Your children are watching you. They are modeling their behavior after you—in areas that you may not even suspect. For example, according to a scientific poll commissioned by CreditCards.com, when adults were asked which family member had the greatest effect on their knowledge of finances and how they managed their money, they most often cited their mothers as being the person with the most influence. And "influence" wasn't necessarily good. If mothers handled their money foolishly, that's what affected their children most. And no, it's not enough to just give lip service to wise money behavior. It was what the mothers actually did with their own money, not what they advised their children to do, that was mirrored by the behavior of their children.

Use Your Unique Qualities to Better the World Around You—Your powerful female brain suits you to work with others to help bring about positive change. Your strong communication skills

and ability to see the bigger picture enable you to bring people together to improve situations. Your greater understanding of others
and ability to empathize makes you caring and compassionate and
able to help your family, your friends, and the larger community.

For example, research out of the University of Cincinnati indicates
that compared to men, women starting new businesses are more likely
to consider individual responsibility and more likely to use their business as a vehicle for social and environmental change. You're always
thinking of others, even while bettering yourself.

This doesn't mean you have to go on the world stage. Just by doing
the tasks that come to you, and taking care of the issues that you face
each day, you can become a positive influence on everyone you meet.

Influence the Men in Your Life to Be Their Best—Your brain is
different from the brains of the men in your life, but by using this
fact, you can begin to understand and communicate with one
another in ways that foster your deeper love and ability to work
together for the good of your relationship and your family.

Research shows that involvement of fathers in the family can be
predicted based on the involvement of mothers, but the reciprocal influence was not significant. It is mothers who can encourage fathers to
be more involved. Help your man by encouraging him to communicate
more effectively, to be more engaged in the life of the family, and to live
a healthier lifestyle.

For you to have this positive effect you need to do everything you
can to make sure that your own brain is healthy and working in top
condition. I call it being a brain warrior for yourself and those you love.
It requires:

- Keeping your brain safe by avoiding toxic foods, chemicals,
  and drugs, and staying away from dangerous activities that
  could traumatize your brain

- Stabilizing your weight at a healthy level
- Getting exercise that keeps your blood flowing—especially to your brain
- Getting sufficient sleep every night, and resolving issues like sleep apnea
- Avoiding bad fats and eating good, healthy fats like olive oil, and omega-3s (through supplements or eating toxin-free fish)
- Keeping your brain flexible and active by exercising it and learning new skills. Did you know your brain actually can grow new neurons? It will if you do your part by feeding it new information and keeping it healthy.
- Resolving issues like ADHD, depression, anxiety, and stress by getting appropriate help. I typically like to start with natural methods before turning to drugs.
- Surrounding yourself with a network of supportive people who will encourage your efforts and help you stay on your healthy program

These things won't happen on their own, and no one will do them for you. You must be conscientious of your own health, biologically, psychologically, socially, and spiritually. Not only is this for your own good, but it is for the good of everyone you influence too.

There's only one time when you can make the necessary changes to boost the power of your brain and improve your health, and that time is right now. Putting it off until tomorrow usually means putting it off indefinitely. How long have you been intending to start living differently? Hasn't it been long enough?

What keeps you from getting started? Is it concerns that you won't succeed? Or not wanting to make the effort? Or thinking it doesn't matter?

I hope that the information in this book has proven to you that you have amazing powers to succeed built right into the very structure of your brain. Your female brain is equipped to understand what you need to do and make connections across your entire brain to call on unexpected resources to help you succeed. You have the ability to love and feel true compassion that can motivate you to achieve great things. Any voice that tells you that you can't do it is just an ANT. Get it out of your life.

How could you not want to make the effort when you can see the problems that arise from not making it? Obesity, toxic exposure, and untreated injuries can lead to decreased quality of life, Alzheimer's disease, and early death. This can't be what you want for yourself and those you love. Make a list of your goals. Post the pictures of the people you love where you can see them every day. Let the love you feel help you get over your initial resistance, and the pleasure of feeling better and better will begin to take over as a powerful motivating factor.

It *does* matter. It matters not only for you but for everyone around you. Women in particular have incredible powers to influence others for the good. Be encouraged by the stories of women everywhere who are beginning to step forward in their societies and are transforming their worlds. What they are doing, you can do.

The world is waiting for you to improve your own corner of life and start a ripple of positive power that can have repercussions far beyond anything you now imagine. To start this beautiful process of transformation, I hope you will take everything that you've learned in this book to unleash the incredibly positive and influential power of your female brain.

GIVE BRAIN HEALTH AWAY

Can one female brain change the world? Yes. I want you to meet my friend Yuk-Lynn from Hong Kong. Yuk-Lynn read a copy of my book *Change Your Brain, Change Your Life*. At the time she was battling low energy, a difficult marriage, and a teenage son who was struggling emotionally and academically. Even though she lived a Pacific Ocean away from one of our clinics, it did not deter her. At first, she sent her husband and son for evaluations, which made a dramatic difference in their lives. Her son, Jonathan, had a hard birth. His scan showed evidence of physical trauma. He told his mom the scan was so helpful. He could see why he was struggling so much. "It's not me," he said. "It was what happened to me." After the scan, he was compliant with the treatment plan and showed significant improvement. Yuk-Lynn's husband, Roy, also helped, which strengthened their marriage. Then Yuk-Lynn came for help, as did her mother, sister, brother, father, and many other family members and friends. She also introduced brain health concepts to her family and friends and has had a huge influence on her community. She and Roy brought together a team of physicians to bring brain SPECT imaging to Hong Kong, in the context of a brain-healthy treatment program. Yuk-Lynn took what she learned and applied it to the good of many other people.

My prayer for you is to do the same. Take this information and pass it on. The world needs your healthy female brain more than ever before.

Hour 12 Exercise—Create Your Own Genius Network

My good friend Joe Polish is a master at relationship building. He has an exercise, "Create Your Own Genius Network," which he generously allowed me to share with you. It can help you thrive and keep you on track toward your goals, in a way similar to that of the small groups at Saddleback. Research has demonstrated that strong relationships are associated with health, happiness, and success. The health of your peer group is one of the strongest predictors of your health and longevity. This exercise will help you create and sustain your own network.

What are your health goals? (Be specific)

1. _____

2. _____

3. _____

4. _____

5. _____

Write down five people who can help you reach your goals and be supportive of your efforts to get and stay healthy:

1. _____

2. _____

3. _____

4. _____

5. _____

Write down exactly how these people can be helpful to you. What wisdom do they have (health advice, exercise buddy, support, etc.)?

1. _____

2. _____

3. _____

4. _____

5. _____

How can you be helpful to them? (Giving back is a key ingredient to making a genius network work.)

1. _____

2. _____

3. _____

4. _____

5. _____

Set aside time each week to connect with the five people in your genius network, whether in person, by phone, or by email or text. If you do this one exercise, you will start to build a great network to help you look better and live a healthier, longer life. Even though this exercise is very simple, it is also powerful. Keep your genius network up-to-date and make sure to support others in their efforts to use their brains to change their health and their lives. You will be supporting yourself in the process.

APPENDIX A:

NATURAL SUPPLEMENTS

To Help You Unleash the Power of Your Female Brain

I'm a great believer in the value of natural supplements. I personally take a handful of supplements every day, and I feel they add significantly to the quality of my life. I recommend them to my family, and I often plan a regimen for my patients based on their individual needs. In my own experience, natural supplements have enhanced the health of my brain while boosting my energy and improving my lab values.

I recommend supplements to my female patients to help with the various issues involved with mood disorders, hormonal imbalances, pregnancy, and the discomforts of perimenopause and menopause. They're also valuable in assuring that developing fetuses receive the building blocks of a healthy body.

Some physicians say that supplements are not necessary if you eat a balanced diet. That would be true if the food we bought in the store had full nutrient value. But does it? As Dr. Mark Hyman wrote in *The Ultra-Mind Solution: Fix Your Broken Brain by Healing Your Body First*, if people "eat wild, fresh, organic, local, non-genetically modified food grown in virgin mineral- and nutrient-rich soils that has not been transported across vast distances and stored for months before being eaten . . . and work and live outside, breathe only fresh unpolluted air, drink only pure, clean water, sleep nine hours a night, move their bodies every day, and are free from chronic stressors and exposure to environmental toxins," then it is possible that they might not need supplements.

But who lives like that? When was the last time you ate an apple that was fresh-picked from the tree? We live in a fast-paced society where we grab food wherever we can get it quickly, skip meals and then fill up on sugar-laden treats and heavily processed foods, and give little thought to eating foods that have been chemically treated. Even if your produce came from an organic farm, it's likely been left on the store shelf (or in your refrigerator) for so long it's lost most of its nutritive value. That's why it's so important to fill in the gaps with a multiple vitamin/mineral supplement.

I like to recommend natural supplements because they can be highly effective, with dramatically fewer side effects than most prescription medications (and usually at significantly less cost). In addition, you don't have to report their use to your insurance company. It's unfortunate, but taking prescription medications can affect your insurability. I know many instances in which people took certain medications and were then were denied or charged higher rates for insurance. Wherever natural alternatives are available, their use should be considered.

But even with my enthusiasm for natural supplements, I must point out that they come with their own set of considerations. First, as great as supplements are, they can't work on their own. They can make a significant difference but only when they are used as part of a complete program whose other elements include a healthy diet, exercise, beneficial thoughts, a supportive peer group, and a wholesome environment.

Also, while they tend to be less expensive than prescription medications, they usually are not covered by insurance, so they can mean more money out of your pocket. And just because something is natural does not mean it is innocuous. Arsenic and cyanide are natural, but they aren't good for you. And natural supplements can have side effects that shouldn't be ignored. For example, St. John's Wort can be a wonderful natural antidepressant, but it can cause sun sensitivity. It can also decrease the effectiveness of a number of medications such as birth control pills. Oh, great! Get depressed, pick up some St. John's Wort from the grocery store, and now you are unexpectedly pregnant. That's not a good solution to depression.

Another major concern about natural supplements is that they often lack quality control. It's very important to use quality brands that you trust. A recommendation from a professional is helpful here, but many people get their supplement advice from the health food store clerk, who may be a summer hire with little background in the field. However, there are supplements available that have been well researched and developed by individuals who are highly knowledgeable and devoted to offering effective, safe products. A little research on your part can help you identify excellent supplements.

Now let's look at how supplements can help with issues that are specific to women.

Help for PMS
- Low progesterone is often one of the causes of PMS symptoms. Progesterone cream used during the last week of a woman's cycle is often helpful.
- In addition, the following supplements can help balance the brain for symptom relief:
  - Calcium citrate (400–500 mg twice a day)
  - Chelated magnesium (200–300 mg twice a day)
  - Vitamin A (5,000 IUs)
  - B complex (with 50 mg of B_6)
  - Evening primrose oil (500 mg twice a day)
  - 5-HTP (50–100 mg twice a day), which may help to boost serotonin and decrease anxiety and worry
  - Green tea or L-tyrosine for focus (500 mg two to three times a day)

• Chasteberry can also help for PMS symptoms, especially breast pain or tenderness, swelling, constipation, irritability, depressed mood or mood alterations, anger, and headache in some women (20–40 mg a day)

Boost Estrogen to Help Relieve Symptoms of Menopause

• Diindolylmethane (DIM) is a phytochemical found in cruciferous vegetables like broccoli and cauliflower. It shifts estrogen metabolism to favor the friendly or harmless estrogen metabolites. DIM can significantly increase the urinary excretion of the "bad" estrogens in as little as four weeks (75–300 mg per day)

• Omega-3 fatty acids (fish oils) contain EPA, which has been reported in laboratory studies to help control estrogen metabolism and decrease the risk of breast cancer. Eating organic beef from grass-fed animals also supplies these fats (2,000 mg per day).

• Calcium D-glucarate is a natural compound found in fruits and vegetables like apples, Brussels sprouts, broccoli, and cabbage. It inhibits the enzyme that contributes to breast, prostate, and colon cancers. It also reduces reabsorbed estrogen from the digestive tract (500–1500 mg per day).

• Probiotics help maintain healthy intestinal flora and healthy estrogen levels. Make sure you get human-strain probiotics that have live cultures (10–60 billion units per day).

• Plant phytoestrogens. The North American Menopause Society specifically recommends dietary isoflavones (found in soy and linseed products), black cohosh, and vitamin E for menopausal symptoms. These plant-based compounds have healthy estrogen-like activity and have been found helpful for a variety of conditions including menopausal symptoms. (They can also help with PMS and may help prevent endometriosis.)

- ° Phytoestrogens are found in many foods. Good sources are nuts and oilseeds (like flaxseed oil), soy, kudzu, red clover, and pomegranate.
- ° Resveratrol is a bioflavonoid antioxidant that occurs naturally in grapes and red wine and has been reported to inhibit breast cancer cell growth in laboratory studies.
- ° Black cohosh is an herb that's been used for centuries by Native Americans for hormonal balance in women. Over the last thirty years, European physicians helping women through menopausal transition have used it extensively. In human studies, black cohosh has been found to decrease hot flashes associated with menopause. Unlike conventional estrogen effects on individuals predisposed to breast cancer, black cohosh has been shown in laboratory studies to inhibit cancer cells. While its long-term safety has not been determined, it seems fine for short-term use. Most studies used 20–80 mg doses twice daily, providing 4–8 mg triterpene glycosides for up to 6 months.

- Melatonin is a hormone produced in the pineal gland that, among other functions, helps us sleep. Melatonin levels decline with age which may lead to the sleep disturbances common during menopause. Melatonin has been shown in laboratory studies to inhibit the growth of breast cancer cells. Melatonin acts as an anti-inflammatory and antioxidant in the brain and other tissues like the intestine. Studies show that low melatonin levels increase breast cancer risk in women. If you are having trouble sleeping, consider taking 3–6 mg melatonin before bed. It may boost your immune system and help you sleep.

- SAMe has also been shown to support healthy joints and decrease pain. The typical dose is anywhere from 400 mg to 800 mg twice a day. It is usually better to take earlier in the day, as it can be energizing. Research suggests you should be cautious with SAMe if you have bipolar disorder.
- There is also interesting new work that shows that DHEA (discussed in the next section) can significantly improve sexual function in menopausal women.

Help for Stress

- DHEA is a natural precursor hormone secreted by the adrenal glands, ovaries, and the brain. It produces estrogen and to a lesser extent, testosterone. DHEA also protects brain cells from the beta-amyloid protein that is associated with Alzheimer's. During periods of chronic stress, the release of the stress hormone cortisol can decrease levels of DHEA, lowering immunity and potentially accelerating the aging processes. Low levels of DHEA have also been linked to weight gain and depression. There is good evidence that validates DHEA supplementation to help support adrenal gland function, mood, and your weight. Generally we start with 10 mg and go up from there. DHEA is usually well tolerated, but there can be some unpleasant side effects like acne and facial hair owing to the tendency of DHEA to increase testosterone levels. These can be avoided by using a specific metabolite of DHEA called 7-Keto-DHEA. It is more expensive than simple DHEA, but it may be preferable in some cases. (The dose of 7-Keto-DHEA is typically 50–100 mg).
- L-theanine (200 mg two or three times a day) for simultaneous relaxation and focus
- Relora (750 mg two to three times a day)

- Magnesium (natural relaxant) (200–300 mg twice a day, especially before bedtime)
- Holy Basil (200–400 mg two to three times a day)
- Ashwagandha (250 mg two to three times a day)
- Rhodiola (200 mg two to three times a day)

LOW TESTOSTERONE LEVELS

There are benefits, besides increased libido, related to testosterone replacement for women, including retention of muscle mass, bone-density retention, improved mood, and reduced cardiovascular risks. Levels of testosterone should be checked in the blood to see if they are low before using any type of bioidentical testosterone or even dietary supplements, such as DHEA.

Before letting your doctor give you testosterone shots or pills, try to boost it naturally by dramatically decreasing or even eliminating sugar, wheat, and processed foods from your diet. A sugar burst has been found to lower testosterone levels by up to 25 percent.

Another way to naturally boost your testosterone level is to start a weight-training program. Building muscle helps your body increase its testosterone levels. The supplements DHEA and zinc can also help. Zinc is necessary to maintain normal testosterone levels. Inadequate zinc levels prevent the pituitary gland from releasing hormones that stimulate testosterone production. Zinc also inhibits the enzyme that converts testosterone into estrogen. If these measures don't work, you may need testosterone replacement.

THYROID

If you have thyroid issues, they can be effectively treated with a number of thyroid medications. Your doctor needs to test your levels regularly to make sure you are not taking too much or too little. There are also a number of natural dietary supplements that support thyroid function, including the herb rosemary, zinc, chromium, potassium, iodine, L-tyrosine, vitamins A, B_2, B_3, B_6, C, D, selenium, seaweed, and ashwagandha. Also, make sure to have healthy testosterone, insulin, and melatonin levels.

INSULIN

- Chromium (200–400 µg) to help balance blood sugar
- Cinnamon (1–6 g; a teaspoon is 4.75 g) to help balance blood sugar

KEY VITAMINS, MINERALS, AND HERBS FOR OVERALL HORMONE BALANCE

For overall good health, I recommend the following supplements for just about everybody:

- Multiple vitamin
- Fish oil (2,000 mg a day)
- Probiotics for gut health to bind bad estrogens (10 to 60 billion CFUs)
- Calcium citrate (400–500 mg twice a day)
- Chelated magnesium (200–300 mg twice a day) to keep your nerves calm
- Vitamin D (2,000 IU of vitamin D daily generally, but it's important to get tested individually) to get the most benefit from calcium
- Zinc (15 mg) for testosterone and thyroid

AMEN SOLUTION SUPPLEMENTS

At the Amen Clinics we make our own line of supplements, the Amen Solution, that have taken over a decade to develop. The reason I developed this line was that I wanted my patients and my own family to have access to the highest quality, research-based supplements available.

Research shows the therapeutic benefit of using supplements to support a healthy mood, sleep, and memory. I strongly recommend that when purchasing a supplement, you consult a health care practitioner familiar with nutritional supplements to determine which supplements and dosages may be most effective for you. Our website (www.amen-clinics.com) contains links to the scientific literature on many different supplements, so you, as a consumer, can be fully informed on the benefits and risks involved. Please remember that supplements can have very powerful effects on the body and caution should be used when combining them with prescription medications.

There are three supplements I typically recommend to *all* of my patients because they are critical to optimal brain function: a multivitamin, fish oil, and vitamin D.

MULTIVITAMINS

According to recent studies, more than 50 percent of Americans do not eat at least five servings of fruits and vegetables a day, the minimum required to get the nutrition you need. In addition, people with weight-management issues often are not eating healthy diets and, as a result, have vitamin and nutrient deficiencies. I recommend that all of my patients take a high-quality multivitamin/mineral complex every day. In an editorial in the *Journal of the American Medical Association*, researchers recommended a daily vitamin for everybody because it helps prevent chronic illness. In addition, people with weight-management issues often are not eating healthy diets and have vitamin and nutrient deficiencies. And research suggests that people who take a multiple vitamin actually have younger-looking DNA.

NeuroVite Plus is the multivitamin we make at the Amen Clinics. It contains a complete range of brain-healthy nutrients. Four capsules a day is the full dose, which contains:

- Vitamin A and high levels of Bs, plus vitamins C, D (2,000 IU), E and K_2
- Minerals—zinc, copper, magnesium, selenium, chromium, manganese, calcium, and magnesium
- Brain nutrients—ALA, acetyl-L-carnitine, and phosphatidyl-serine
- Equivalent nutrients to:
    - 1 apple (quercitin)
    - 1 tomato (lycopene)
    - 1 serving fresh spinach (lutein)
    - 1 serving broccoli (broccoli seed concentrate)
    - 2 L red wine (resveratrol, without the alcohol)
    - 1 cup blueberries (pterostilbene)
- A full dose of a stabilized probiotic

FISH OIL

For years, I have been writing about the benefits of omega-3 fatty acids, which are found in fish oil supplements. I personally take a fish oil supplement every day and recommend that *all* of my patients do the same. Research has found that omega-3 fatty acids are essential for optimal brain and body health.

For example, according to researchers at the Harvard School of Public Health, having low levels of omega-3 fatty acids is one of the leading preventable causes of death and has been associated with heart disease, strokes, depression, suicidal behavior, ADD, dementia, and obesity. There is also scientific evidence that low levels of omega-3 fatty acids play a role in weight control.

Research in the last few years has also revealed that diets rich in omega-3 fatty acids help promote a healthy emotional balance and positive mood in later years, possibly because DHA is a main component of the brain's synapses. A growing body of scientific evidence indicates that fish oil helps ease symptoms of depression. One twenty-year study involving 3,317 men and women found that people with the highest consumption of EPA and DHA were less likely to have symptoms of depression. Omega-3 fatty acids have also been shown to benefit cognitive performance at every age.

My recommendation for most adults is to take between 1 and 2 g high-quality fish oil a day balanced between EPA and DHA.

Omega-3 Power is our brand to support healthy brain and heart function by providing highly purified omega-3 fatty acids (EPA and DHA) from the most advanced production, detoxification, and purification process in the industry. It is produced under the natural product industry's most rigorous standards. Each batch of our oil is independently analyzed by the third-party lab Eurofins for more than 250 environmental contaminants, including PCBs. Oil is certified to be over twenty times lower than California's Proposition 65 requirement of less than 90 nanograms per day. Our brand also exceeds all other domestic and international regulatory standards. Two softgels contain 2.8 grams of fish oil, and 860mg of EPA and 580mg of DHA.

VITAMIN D

Vitamin D, also known as the sunshine vitamin, is best known for building bones and boosting the immune system. But it is also an essential vitamin for brain health, mood, memory, and your weight. While classified as a vitamin, it is a steroid hormone vital to health. Low levels of vitamin D have been associated with depression, autism, psychosis, Alzheimer's disease, multiple sclerosis, heart disease, diabetes, cancer, and obesity. Unfortunately, vitamin D deficiencies are becoming more and more common, in part because we are spending more time indoors and using more sunscreen.

Vitamin D is so important to brain function that its receptors can be found throughout the brain. Vitamin D plays a critical role in many of the most basic cognitive functions, including learning and making memories. These are just some of the areas where vitamin D affects how well your brain works, according to a 2008 review that appeared in the *FASEB Journal*.

The lower your vitamin D levels, the more likely you are to feel blue rather than happy. Low levels of vitamin D have long been associated with a higher incidence of depression. In recent years, we've seen evidence that vitamin D supplementation can improve moods.

The current recommended dose for vitamin D is 400 IU daily, but most experts agree that this is well below the physiological needs of most individuals and instead suggest 2,000 IU of vitamin D daily. I think it is very important to test your individual needs, especially if you are overweight or obese since your body may not absorb the vitamin D as efficiently if you are heavier. Our vitamin D_3, comes as 1,000 IU tablets, 2,000 IU tablets, or as 10,000 IU liquid.

BRAIN AND MEMORY POWER BOOST

This is the supplement formulated to help in our brain enhancement work with active and retired NFL players. When used in conjunction with a brain-healthy program, we demonstrated significant improvement in memory, reasoning, attention, processing speed, and accuracy. It was so effective that I take it every day.

Brain and Memory Power Boost includes the super-antioxidant N-acetylcysteine (NAC), along with phosphatidylserine to maintain the integrity of cell membranes, huperzine A and acetyl-L-carnitine to enhance acetylcholine availability, and vinpocetine and ginkgo biloba to enhance blood flow. This is a novel combination of powerful antioxidants and nutrients essential in enhancing and protecting brain health. It supports overall brain health, circulation, memory, and concentration.

CRAVING CONTROL

The key to successful weight management is eating a brain-healthy diet and managing your cravings. In support of this goal, Craving Control was developed, a powerful new nutritional supplement formulated to support healthy blood sugar and insulin levels while providing antioxidants and nutrients to the body. Our formulation includes NAC and glutamine to reduce cravings, chromium and ALA to support stable blood sugar levels and a brain-healthy chocolate and DL-phenylalanine designed to boost endorphins.

This is the formula we use at the Amen Clinics in our own weight-loss groups. In the first group, participants who used the craving formula and attended each group, lost an average of 10 pounds in ten weeks.

RESTFUL SLEEP

Sleep is essential to healthy brain function. Restful Sleep is formulated with a combination of nutrients designed to support a calm mind and promote a deep, relaxed, restful night's sleep. This supplement contains both immediate and time-released melatonin to keep you asleep throughout the entire night, plus the calming neurotransmitter GABA, a combination of the essential elements zinc and magnesium, and the herb valerian, which together may produce an overall sedative effect to help support sleep. At the Amen Clinics we refer to Restful Sleep as "the hammer" because so many people have told us it has helped them.

SAMe Mood and Movement Support

SAMe has scientific research suggesting it helps support mood, movement, and pain control. It is intimately involved in the creation of the key neurotransmitters, serotonin, dopamine, and norepinephrine that support healthy mood. And as an added advantage, SAMe has also been shown to support healthy joints and decrease pain. The typical dose is 400–800 mg twice a day. It is usually better to take earlier in the day, as it can be energizing. Research suggests you should be cautious with SAMe if you have bipolar disorder.

SEROTONIN MOOD SUPPORT

Serotonin Mood Support promotes normal serotonin levels by providing 5-HTP, a direct precursor to serotonin, along with a proprietary extract of saffron, shown clinically to support a normal mood. Vitamin B$_6$ and inositol are included to provide additional synergistic support. Serotonin Mood Support is useful to support a healthy mood when serotonin levels are suspected to be low. It seems to be especially helpful for people who tend to get stuck on negative thoughts or negative behaviors. It has also been shown to help support healthy sleep patterns.

FOCUS AND ENERGY OPTIMIZER

Formulated without caffeine that makes people jittery, Focus and Energy Optimizer supports both focus and healthy energy levels. It is formulated with green tea and choline to help with focus, along with three powerful adaptogens, which act synergistically to enhance endurance and stamina. The adaptogens ashwaganda, rhodiola, and panax ginseng have been scientifically shown to improve the body's resistance to stress and support a healthy immune system.

GABA CALMING SUPPORT

GABA Calming Support promotes natural relaxation and calm by providing a combination of inhibitory neurotransmitters vital to quieting an overactive mind. It contains clinically tested and natural Pharma GABA, shown to promote relaxation by increasing calming, focused brain waves while also reducing other brain waves associated with worry. Complimenting this clinically tested and natural substance are vitamin B$_6$, magnesium, and lemon balm, an herb traditionally known for its calming effects.

NOTE ON REFERENCES

The information in *Unleash the Power of the Female Brain* is based on more than 250 references and sources, including scientific studies, books, interviews with medical experts, statistics from government agencies and health organizations, and other reliable resources. Printed out, the references take up many pages. In an effort to save a few trees, I have decided to place them exclusively on the www.amenclinics.com website. I invite you to view them at www.amenclinics.com/unleashthepowerofthefemalebrain.

ACKNOWLEDGMENTS

I am grateful to the many people who have helped me with this work. I am especially grateful to all of my patients and friends who have allowed me to share their stories with you, especially my wonderful wife, Tana. I am grateful to Dr. James LaValle and Dr. Tami Meraglia for their guidance and insights. I am grateful to Dee Eastman, director of the Daniel Plan at Saddleback Church, for her insights. I am also grateful to my many friends and colleagues at Saddleback for their love and support. Joe Polish: Thank you, my friend, for creating the "Create Your Own Genius Network" exercise and allowing me to pass it along to our readers.

Dr. Ellen Dickstein and Rachel Krantz were invaluable in the process of researching, interviewing, and completing this book. Our research department, including Dr. Kristen Willeumeir and Derek Taylor, provided valuable insights and encouragement. Other staff at Amen Clinics, Inc., as always, provided tremendous help and support during this process, especially my personal assistant, Catherine Hanlon; our medical director of our Washington, D.C., clinic, Dr. Joseph Annibali; our general manager for Amen Clinics, Susan Haeger; our general manager for MindWorks, Bernie Landes; our director of marketing, Murray Brannen; and our publicity director, David Jar.

I also wish to thank my amazing literary team at Crown Archetype, especially my kind and thoughtful editor, Julia Pastore, and my publisher, Tina Constable. I am grateful, as always, to my literary agent, Faith Hamlin, along with Stefanie Diaz, our foreign rights agent. If you are reading this outside of the United States, Stefanie made that happen. In addition, I am grateful to all of my friends and colleagues at public television stations across the country. Public television is a treasure to our country and I am grateful to be able to partner with stations to bring our message of hope and healing to you. I love all of you.

ABOUT DANIEL G. AMEN, M.D.

Dr. Amen is a physician, psychiatrist, teacher, and five time *New York Times* bestselling author. He is widely regarded as one of the world's foremost experts on applying brain imaging science to clinical psychiatric practice. He is a board-certified child and adult psychiatrist and a Distinguished Fellow of the American Psychiatric Association. He is the medical director of Amen Clinics, Inc., in Newport Beach and San Francisco, California; Bellevue, Washington; Reston, Virginia; Atlanta, Georgia; and New York. Amen Clinics have the world's largest database of functional brain scans relating, totaling nearly eighty thousand scans on patients from ninety countries.

Dr. Amen is widely regarded as a gifted teacher, taking complex concepts in neuropsychiatry, neuroimaging, and brain health and making them easily accessible to other professionals and the general public.

Dr. Amen is the lead researcher on the world's largest brain imaging/brain rehabilitation study on professional football players, which not only demonstrated significant brain damage in a high percentage of retired players but also the possibility for rehabilitation in many with the principles that underlie his work.

Under the direction of Pastor Rick Warren, Dr. Amen, together with Drs. Mark Hyman and Mehmet Oz, is one of the chief architects on Saddleback Church's Daniel Plan, a fifty-two-week program to get churches physically, emotionally, and spiritually healthy.

Dr. Amen is the author of fifty professional articles; the coauthor of the chapter "Functional Imaging in Clinical Practice" in the Comprehensive Textbook of Psychiatry; and the author of thirty books, including *Change Your Brain, Change Your Life*; *Magnificent Mind at Any Age*;

Change Your Brain, Change Your Body; *The Amen Solution*; and *Use Your Brain to Change Your Age*. He is also the author of *Healing ADD, Making a Good Brain Great, Healing the Hardware of the Soul* and coauthor of *Unchain Your Brain, Healing Anxiety and Depression,* and *Preventing Alzheimer's*.

Dr. Amen is the producer and star of six highly popular shows about the brain, which have raised more than forty-four million dollars for public television.

A small sample of the organizations Dr. Amen has spoken for include the National Security Agency; the National Science Foundation; Harvard's Learning and the Brain Conference; Franklin Covey; the National Council of Juvenile and Family Court Judges; and the Supreme Courts of Delaware, Ohio, and Wyoming. Dr. Amen's work has been featured in *Newsweek, Parade,* the *New York Times Magazine, Men's Health,* and *Cosmopolitan*.

Dr. Amen is married to Tana; he is the father of four children, and grandfather to Elias, Julian, Angelina, Emmy, and Liam. He is an avid table tennis player.

ABOUT AMEN CLINICS, INC.

Amen Clinics, Inc. (ACI) was established in 1989 by Daniel G. Amen, M.D. It specializes in innovative diagnosis and treatment planning for a wide variety of behavioral, learning, emotional, cognitive, and weight problems for children, teenagers, and adults. ACI has an international reputation for evaluating brain-behavior problems, such as ADD, depression, anxiety, school failure, brain trauma, obsessive-compulsive disorders, aggressiveness, marital conflict, cognitive decline, brain toxicity from drugs or alcohol, and obesity.

Brain SPECT imaging is performed in the Amen Clinics. ACI has the world's largest database of brain scans for emotional, cognitive, and behavioral problems. ACI welcomes referrals from physicians, psychologists, social workers, marriage and family therapists, drug and alcohol counselors, and individual patients.

Amen Clinics, Inc., Newport Beach
4019 Westerly Pl., Suite 100
Newport Beach, CA 92660
(888) 564- 2700

Amen Clinics, Inc., San Francisco
1000 Marina Blvd, Suite 100
Brisbane, CA 94005
(888) 564- 2700

Amen Clinics, Inc., Northwest
616 120th Ave. NE, Suite C100
Bellevue, WA 98005
(888) 564–2700

Amen Clinics, Inc., DC
1875 Campus Commons Dr.
Reston, VA 20191
(888) 564- 2700

Amen Clinics New York
16 E. Fortieth St., 9th Floor
New York, NY 10016
(888) 564- 2700

Amen Clinics Atlanta
5901-C Peachtree Dunwoody Rd. NE, Suite 65
Atlanta, GA 30328
(888) 564–2700

WWW.AMENCLINICS.COM

Amenclinic.com is an educational, interactive website geared toward mental health and medical professionals, educators, students, and the general public. It contains a wealth of information and resources to help you learn about and optimize your brain. The site contains more than three hundred color brain SPECT images, thousands of scientific abstracts on brain SPECT imaging for psychiatry, a free brain-healthy audit, and much, much more.

WWW.THEAMENSOLUTION.COM

Based on Dr. Amen's thirty years as a clinical psychiatrist, he has developed a sophisticated online community to hold your hand to get thinner, smarter and happier, and younger. It includes:

- Detailed questionnaires, to help you know your brain type and personalize program to your own needs
- Interactive daily journal to track your numbers, calories, and brain-healthy habits
- Hundreds of brain-healthy recipes, tips, shopping lists, and menu plans
- An exclusive, award-winning 24/7 Brain Gym membership
- Daily tips, even text messages, to help you remember your supplements and stay on track
- A relaxation room to help you eliminate stress and overcome negative thinking patterns
- Plus much, much more (www.theamensolution.com)